℞ Fitness for Weight Loss

The Medically Sound Solution to Get Fit and Save Your Life

JULIA KARLSTAD, M.ED.
Certified Physical Fitness Specialist
Certified Strength and Conditioning Specialist

Copyright © 2009 Julia Karlstad
All rights reserved.

ISBN: 1-4392-3413-2
ISBN-13: 9781439234136

Visit www.booksurge.com to order additional copies.

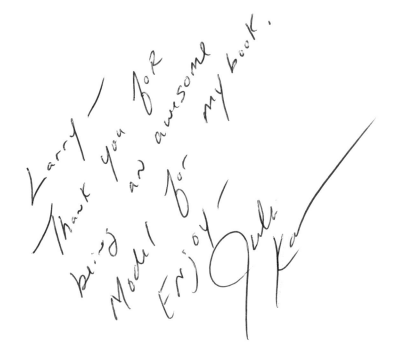

This book is dedicated to people everywhere who desire to become physically fit, lose weight, and make a positive change in their lives to look better, feel better, and live longer. It is also dedicated to health and fitness professionals who want to gain more knowledge in order to physically train and educate people to overcome physical limitations or medical conditions in an effort to get fit, lose weight, and live a healthier life.

Contents

- About the Author IX
- Preface XI
- Acknowledgments XIII

Part I. Committing to an Exercise Program and Preparing to Begin

Chapter 1. Embracing a Lifestyle Change. 3
- Using the Past without Getting Stuck   3
- Accepting Change   5
- Setting Goals   6

Chapter 2. Finding the Motivation to Move Your Body. 9
- Benefits of Exercise   9
- Not "Buying Into" Buying the "Magic Pill"   14
- Getting Motivated to Exercise   15
- Recognizing Obstacles   16
- Overcoming Obstacles   17
- Finding and Working with a Qualified Fitness Professional   26

Chapter 3. Creating Comfort in Your Fitness Regimen 29
- Workout Locations (Environments)   30
- Workout Attire and Gear   36
- Takeaway Points on Exercise Comfort   41

Part II. Initiating and Maintaining an Exercise Program

Chapter 4. Understanding and Building 45
on the Four Pillars of Fitness

Flexibility (Stretching) Exercises	46
Cardiovascular Exercise	47
Strength (Resistance) Training	48
Healthy Diet	49
Weight-Loss Surgery Dietary Guidelines	56
Sample Weight-Loss Diet	57

Chapter 5. Getting Started with Exercise 59

Rules of Thumb	62
Cardio Exercise	63
Strength Training	64
Flexibility Exercises	65
Dietary and Hydration Guidelines	66

Chapter 6. Understanding and Accepting Your Limitations: .. 67
Exercising Without Injury

Rules of Thumb	68
Arthritis	69
Breast Cancer	70
Cancer (All)	71
Diabetes	72
Fibromyalgia	76
Heart Disease	77
Hip or Knee Replacement	78
Hypertension (High Blood Pressure)	79
Lumbar or Cervical Back Problems	81

Lumbar or Cervical Disc Disease (Spondylosis, Disc Herniation, Bulging Disc, or Spinal Stenosis) ... 82
Multiple Sclerosis ... 82
Muscular Dystrophy ... 83
Obesity in Adults ... 84
Obesity in Children ... 86
Osteoporosis/Osteopenia ... 88
Pregnancy ... 89
Shoulder Injury ... 92
Weight-Loss (Bariatric) Surgery: Gastric Bypass, LAP-BAND, Gastric Sleeve, or Duodenal Switch. ... 92
Wheelchair Bound or Amputee ... 96

Chapter 7. Maximizing Your Body's Fat-Burning Capacity .. 103
Fuel Sources ... 103
VO2 Max Testing to Determine Target Heart Rate ... 109
Karvonen Method to Determine Target Heart Rate ... 112

Chapter 8. Performing Fitness Assessments and Reassessments . 117
Overall Health-Related Assessments ... 118
Posture and Balance Assessments ... 124
Body Weight, Height, Body Mass Index, and Body Composition ... 128
Girth Measurements ... 134
Laboratory Work-up ... 141
Flexibility Assessments ... 144
Cardiovascular Assessments ... 157
Muscular Strength Assessments ... 164

Part III. Going the "Extra Mile" to Get Results

Chapter 9. Doctors' Keys to Successful Weight Loss 177
A Bariatrician's Perspective — 177
A Bariatric Surgeon's Perspective (by Lloyd Stegemann) — 184
A Psychologist's Perspective — 188

Chapter 10. Client Testimonials 205
Michelle Tallon — 206
Kim Oerkfitz — 210
Stefanie Alvheim — 217
Meg Lesieur — 219

Appendix A. Recommendations for Workout Apparel, ... 223
Accessories, and Equipment

Appendix B. Rate of Perceived Exertion (RPE): 225
How Hard You Feel You Are Exercising

Glossary 227

Index 245

About the Author

Julia Karlstad has a Master of Education degree in exercise science as well as a Bachelor of Science degree in basic sciences from the U.S. Air Force Academy. She also holds two nationally recognized fitness certifications: Strength and Conditioning Specialist from the National Strength and Conditioning Association and Physical Fitness Specialist from The Cooper Institute. In addition, she is an active member of the American College of Sports Medicine, the National Strength and Conditioning Association, and the Obesity Action Coalition.

Julia has helped people lose weight for many years. She has worked with thousands of clients, including a 600-pound individual, an 82-year-old, a 9-year-old pushing 200 pounds, pre- and post-weight-loss surgery clients, wheelchair-bound individuals, soldiers, athletes, and marathon runners. She worked in a medically supervised weight-loss clinic for three years. She developed and directed the exercise physiology department for a bariatric program that consisted of two bariatric hospitals and three medically supervised weight-loss clinics. In addition, she has managed a multidisciplinary medical and surgical weight-loss clinic consisting of a full fitness center, medical clinic, sleep labs, nutrition unit, and patient education programs. She recently founded JKFITNESS and manages all aspects of this health and fitness company.

JULIA'S TESTIMONIAL:

I am passionate about helping people. There is no better feeling than positively changing someone's life. I've celebrated the accomplishments of many of my clients. Whether their goals were losing 5 lb or 300 lb, being able to conceive or adopt a child, being able to play with their children, bending over to tie their shoes, getting out of their wheelchairs, getting rid of their walkers, avoiding knee-replacement surgery or preparing for knee-replacement surgery, preparing for weight-loss surgery, recovering from an injury, becoming more ambulatory, getting off their medications, being able to mow their lawn, being able to go to the grocery store by themselves, climbing stairs, hiking, jogging for the first time or being able to travel, there is no better feeling than celebrating these accomplishments with them.

Helping people accomplish their health and weight-loss goals through exercise is much more rewarding than helping someone run faster or jump higher. I've helped people who are severely overweight to obese and suffer from physical and medical limitations "get their lives back." Now that is gratifying! I trust that by reading this book and committing to a life of fitness your life will be transformed and enriched.

Preface

The main purpose of this book is to inform, educate, and provide functional yet realistic guidance for the overweight to obese who have always struggled with their weight. However, anyone seeking a higher level of fitness and optimal health will also find it invaluable. One of the first steps in making a commitment to achieving physical fitness and optimal weight loss is to understand that weight management is a lifestyle habit. In order to be successful with individual weight-loss goals, one must commit to a routine exercise regimen and constantly monitor his/her dietary intake.

Most people know that controlling their weight means watching their diet and doing some form of exercise. The challenge lies in finding the answer on how to get fit. Many articles you read, television specials you hear, and personal trainers in mainstream gyms do not have the expertise to guide you down a successful, long-term weight-management path. This book gives you a comprehensive approach on how to exercise to lose weight for good and optimize your health.

I rarely see a magazine cover without an article referring to weight loss, healthy eating tips, or the perfect get slim workout. Popular headlines include "Melt the Last 10 Pounds," "Slim, Firm, & Tone," "Get Fit Anywhere," "Fast Healthy Meal Ideas and Recipes," and "Your Easy 20-Minute Workout." These headlines grab your attention because you want to know how to get fit quickly. Some of the articles are great, but most give you only a fraction of what you really need to know to be successful.

This book describes a specific exercise program to lose excess weight and become physically fit as well as specific dietary guidelines, including some sample menus. Readers will learn an all-inclusive approach to exercise from someone who is formally educated and experienced in dealing with exercise specific to weight loss. They will also learn exactly how to exercise not only to maximize fat loss, but also to lose weight long term and injury free.

In short, this book peels back the layers of fitness so that every person, no matter what fitness level, will thoroughly understand how to exercise in order to achieve lasting weight loss and an optimal level of fitness. It also includes exercise guidelines for specific medical conditions and limitations. Regardless of your current health and fitness condition, after reading this book you'll know how to get started, stay committed, and exercise injury free.

The book is divided into three major parts: Part I, Committing to an Exercise Program and Preparing to Begin, Part II, Initiating and Maintaining an Exercise Program, and Part III, Going the "Extra Mile" to Get Results. Part III provides keys to successful weight loss from Dr. Tamyra Rogers, a physician practicing in the field of medicine concerned with weight loss (a bariatrician); Dr. Lloyd Stegemann, a weight-loss surgeon; and Dr. Edward Wilks, a licensed psychologist; and testimonials from some of my clients who have worked with me as their personal trainer.

It is very important to understand that before you start any exercise program, you should consult with your physician. The information in this book is not intended as medical advice. All information is accurate to the author's best knowledge, and publications and other resources used are considered authoritative. Information herein is not intended to diagnose or recommend treatment for any disease. This book is intended solely to educate readers about fitness and motivate them to be physically active and lose excess weight. The outcome of any actions suggested in this book are the sole responsibility of the person taking these actions.

JK

Acknowledgments

I want to thank God for giving me the gift of compassion and empathy for people. I also give gratitude to the Lord for giving me the desire to pass along my knowledge in an effort to make a positive impact on people's lives. This book would not have been complete without the love and support of my family. My sincere gratitude to my mother and father, Carolyn and Dennis Karlstad, for giving me the strength to follow my dreams. To my sister, Heather, many thanks for believing in all that I take on.

My closest and beloved friend, Mary Ambrose, deserves very special recognition. She personally supported me from start to finish with this book, and her sacrifices along the way did not go unnoticed.

I also give tribute to all the clients I have worked with over the years. I have enjoyed every moment with them and have learned a tremendous amount as I've witnessed numerous individuals make the change of a lifetime. Special credit goes to Kim Oerkfitz, Michelle Tallon, Meg Lesieur, Stefanie Alvheim, Carolyn Smiser, Tim Maloney and Elva Jumper for sharing their health and weight-loss testaments.

I am indebted to the many professionals in the field of bariatrics who I have had the opportunity to work with over the years. The doctors, surgeons, dieticians, nurses, fitness professionals, and psychologists have all helped me truly understand the overweight-to-obese client. In a concerted effort, we have all helped fight the obesity epidemic. Many thanks to Dr. Rogers, Dr. Stegemann, and Dr. Wilks for helping me create the chapter Doctor's Keys to Successful Weight Loss. I am also grateful for Nichole Ulibarri's contribution of the sample weight loss menu as well as her review of the dietary guidelines for healthy weight loss.

I want to thank my editor, Kathleen O'Brien. She was patient with me in the authorship of my first book. Her attention to detail and consistent follow-up were paramount in seeing this book to publication and print. I thank Mark

Oerkfitz, my photographer, who was extremely patient in spending numerous hours to ensure the best pictures were portrayed in my book. High five to my close friend, Megan Thiedeman, for helping me clean up the finer points of my book. I am also appreciative to Alicia LePray, Larry Thiedeman, Yvette Martinez, Mary Ambrose and Melissa Barker for being such wonderful models for all of the pictures utilized throughout the book. I give tribute to my graphic designer, Bruce Coderre. His creative talent helped bring my book to life. My sincere gratitude also goes to Phyllis May and Trish Maloney; they both helped mentor me along the path of authorship.

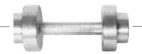

Part I

COMMITTING TO AN EXERCISE PROGRAM AND PREPARING TO BEGIN

Chapter 1
Embracing a Lifestyle Change

USING THE PAST WITHOUT GETTING STUCK

If you are overweight or obese, it is important to sit back and reflect. How did I get to this point? Am I really this big? Is this really who I am? How did this happen? Why didn't I realize I was becoming this overweight? Have you asked yourself these questions lately? Or, have you engaged in the following self-talk? "I used to be in really good shape; I just don't understand how I let myself go this far. I just didn't see it until my weight began to limit my daily activities. My weight is starting to interfere with my social activities as well as with my family and responsibilities at work."

Maybe your excess weight has put you out of a job completely. Have you heard yourself making remarks like the following? "I was always overweight as a child. My siblings were overweight and so were my parents and grandparents. I really didn't have a hope. I just haven't taken care of myself." "Everyone and everything else in my life has taken precedence over me…my kids, my family, my job. I feel guilty any time I do try to do things for myself, such as exercise. Everything I do revolves around food. I feel like I have no control anymore. Often, I use food to comfort me in times of stress or when I'm feeling down. I just haven't been disciplined. My life is so hectic and I'm always eating out. I frequently stop and get fast food because it is easier. I don't have time to eat healthy and exercise; it's too much work."

Does your weight strain your relationships with family and friends? Have you heard yourself making remarks like the following? "I've tried to lose weight, but it seems like my closest family members and friends always sabotage my efforts.

I lose 20 or 30 lb and my family and friends don't support me. They ask me why I'm doing this and tell me I really don't need to lose weight, or they simply tell me that it's not going to work."

Or, maybe your family and friends are the opposite—they constantly nag you about your weight and make you feel insecure and depressed. They talk about how you need to do something about your weight and sometimes even make offensive comments regarding your size. Have you found yourself saying anything like the following to yourself or others? "I thought these people loved me. Why are they hurting me like this? I have always been known as the 'fat friend' . . . it's a part of my social status. My friends and family have labeled me as this and I've accepted it. I'm afraid to lose weight for fear of losing my identity along with some of my friends."

Have you tried to lose weight but failed? Have you heard yourself making remarks like the following? "I never really noticed I was putting on so much weight. When I looked at myself in the mirror, I still felt like I was looking at the old me. It wasn't until I saw a photo of myself when it hit me. I couldn't believe that was me. I've tried every single diet, exercise, and weight loss program and every time I fail. Diet pills, herbal supplements, Weight Watchers, life-time member at the local gym, Atkin's, South Beach Diet, Jenny Craig, and Curves. I lose some weight while I'm on one of those programs and then I gain it back. In fact, I would say I'm pretty good at losing weight; the problem is keeping it off. Sometimes, I gain back more than I lost. It has been a never-ending battle that I never win. Nothing seems to work for me in the long term."

Reflecting on the past and truly identifying what caused you to become overweight or obese will start you down the path to overcoming your obstacles. Obstacles are discussed in detail in a subsequent chapter, but it is important to recognize obstacles so that you can focus on your goals instead of the obstacles. This style of thinking will help you persevere in order to accept the lifestyle changes you are about to make.

Now, let's talk exercise as it relates to you. Some of the answers to the questions above may be attributable to a lack of physical activity or exercise in your life. Even though you are in a period of reflection, remember not to harbor the past. It is now time to look toward the future and begin your new lifestyle. Simply learn from your mistakes and do your best to avoid making the same mistakes again. Don't believe that just because you failed in the past that you will automatically fail again. Use a different approach and *do not give up*.

ACCEPTING CHANGE

The next problem you may be struggling with is accepting change. Change is very difficult for many people. Many of us find comfort in some of our good and not-so-good habits. Maybe you are afraid to change because you fear giving up these comforts. It's okay and natural to be afraid and uncomfortable with a lifestyle change. Changing old habits isn't easy; many people find it hard to adjust to change.

Take a moment to think about the habits in your life that need to change—specifically the habits that have most contributed to your weight gain over the years. Write down these habits in the spaces below.

HABITS THAT HAVE CONTRIBUTED TO MY WEIGHT GAIN:

1. _____
2. _____
3. _____
4. _____
5. _____

If you think about it, many of these actions or inactions are self-destructive. The more we eat the things we shouldn't eat, drink the things we shouldn't drink, and continue to be less and less physically active, the more we harm ourselves. Take food for example: Food is meant for survival, yet many people live to eat rather than eating to live. When you continuously eat more food than your system really needs, you are essentially poisoning yourself in a manner similar to overdosing on a medication or drinking too much alcohol. Your body is designed to take in only a certain amount of food. In addition, when you choose to eat processed, fried, or trans-fatty foods, you're adding fuel to the fire. Your organs, muscles, and brain do not want to use this type of food for fuel. Essentially, you are putting toxic gas into your system, which, over time, will bog it down. The same goes for exercise. The less you exercise, the more lethargic your body becomes. The human body "wants" to be active. The less you move, the more you harm your body in the long run because it will be less efficient at burning fat, which will ultimately result in excess weight on your body's frame. This excess weight can lead to heart failure, joint problems, diabetes, high cholesterol, arthritis, and respiratory complications. If you want to stop harming your body, make changes today. These changes will put you on the path of weight-loss success and prevent the poisoning effects of excessive food intake and eating foods that are harmful.

SETTING GOALS

Now that you've identified some of the habits that have contributed to your weight gain, think about how you're going to change these habits. Change can be significantly easier if you set realistic goals. So, be sure your goals are realistic. I emphasize *goals*, plural. Set more than one goal and make sure that each goal is attainable. Goals are important: If you don't know where you are going, you will not know how to get there.

In addition to setting goals, you should create a timeline, do some initial assessments, and repeatedly monitor your progress. Monitoring your progress is critical because if you don't know where you started and how you did along the way, you will have no idea how far you've come. This solidifies the need to set goals. Once you've set your goals, the next step is making sure you document your progress. If you are willing to work through the initial discomfort, you will begin to gain more confidence to follow through with the lifestyle changes you've decided to make. Just remember, your changes may need to be gradual. Take a moment to write down your goals.

MY GOALS INCLUDE:

1. _____
2. _____
3. _____
4. _____
5. _____

IDENTIFY YOUR TWO MOST IMPORTANT GOALS AND FILL IN YOUR TIMELINE TO ACHIEVE THESE GOALS:

1. I'd like to achieve goal number _____ in _____ (days/weeks/months/years).
2. I'd like to achieve goal number _____ in _____ (days/weeks/months/years).

As you make changes to live a healthier lifestyle and as you start to incorporate regular physical activity into your life, be proud of the changes you make. Take each day one step at a time. Sometimes, you just need to take baby steps. Before you know it, you'll see considerable progress. When you achieve each daily success, you will find comfort in the balance of food, activity, and your overall attitude toward the "new you."

Control what you can control and do your best not to worry about things you have no control over. With regard to fitness, you control your decision to be physically active. You might think you don't have enough time, but you have to *make* time. Treat your exercise time as your own "sacred time" or necessary time like a doctor's appointment. Remember to ask yourself this question, "Which is better: to exercise one hour a day or risk death 24 hours a day?" I think you know the answer. This may seem like an extreme or exaggerated statement, but exercise and physical activity have been proved to decrease the mortality rate. Most important, exercise is a critical component to successful long-term weight loss.

It is imperative to understand that fitness is a life-long endeavor, not a single destination. Some say fitness is a journey, but this saying implies an ending or stopping point. You must always continue to stay physically active in order to accomplish long-term weight management. In order to change your lifestyle, you must change the way you live, and if exercise has been challenging for you, this book will help you get started and stay committed.

Perhaps you are thinking, "Okay, I understand my need to exercise, but I really hate exercising. If I liked it, I probably wouldn't be in this situation." The good news is that you don't have to "kill" yourself in order to be fit and lose weight. Exercise doesn't have to be a bad or difficult experience; in fact, starting out slowly and then gradually progressing is a good thing. Keep in mind that exercise is stress on your body. Fortunately, it can be *good* stress, provided you "introduce" exercise to your body in an appropriate way. If you don't begin exercising in an appropriate manner or don't exercise properly, the stress may cause negative effects and sabotage your weight-loss efforts in a manner similar to how you become run down or physically ill when there is too much stress in your life.

More exercise is not always better exercise. In fact, your body burns fat more efficiently if exercise is done at a low-to-moderate level of intensity. This is discussed in greater detail in Chapter 7. The key is exercising smarter, not harder. The main objective is to exercise so that you maximize your body's ability to burn fat. If every time you exercise you remember to think, "I'm creating a body that is really efficient at burning fat; this is helping me to lose weight faster and more easily," changing your activity level can be a very rewarding and positive experience.

Now that you are ready to change, the next chapter outlines (1) how you can motivate yourself to start exercising and (2) how to overcome obstacles to exercising that may arise along the way. If you understand these as well as how to exercise and are able to maintain a regular, consistent physical fitness regimen, you are on the road to long-term weight-management success.

Chapter 2
Finding the Motivation to Move Your Body

Motivating yourself to exercise is probably one of the most difficult things to master. I do not know many people who *love* to exercise, and even if they say they do, they are probably referring to the euphoric effect they get after exercise versus the actual act of exercising. Even top-level athletes struggle to find the motivation to practice their skills and push themselves to become more and more physically fit. This being said, it is normal to struggle because of a lack of motivation at times. Knowing how to overcome that lack of motivation and start moving is the true test.

BENEFITS OF EXERCISE

Let's start by reviewing the benefits of exercise. You've probably heard of most, if not all, of these benefits before, but it is important to review all of them.

WEIGHT LOSS

Since the main objective is weight loss, let's review the benefits of exercise that cumulatively result in weight loss. Exercise increases daily caloric expenditure, facilitates weight loss, decreases body fat, decreases inches, increases fat-free body mass, and increases the body's fat-burning capacity. You want to lose weight, right? These six benefits will help you do just that! Let me expand on each of these benefits a bit further so that you can begin to realize how your body works physiologically when you exercise:

- Increasing your daily caloric expenditure is probably the one benefit that most directly affects your weight loss. The following points give details about the ways that exercise increases your daily caloric expenditure.

- The most obvious caloric expenditure is that your body requires more calories to function when you are more physically active. Think of your body as a car: The more you drive your "car"—that is, the more physically active you are—the more fuel you have to put in it. Increased physical activity, in turn, increases your metabolism and the number of calories burned in one day. Simply put, your body will burn more calories per minute when you are active than when you are sedentary.
- How many and what type of calories you burn while exercising depends on the level of intensity at which you work. Understand that exercise allows your body to burn fat better. The more fit you become, the better your body burns fat, thus the easier it is to lose weight and ultimately maintain the weight loss long term.
- So how many calories can be burned? A person's physical activity throughout the day can account for approximately 20-25 percent of the total calories burned in one day. The majority of your daily caloric expenditure comes from your resting metabolic rate (RMR). Your RMR is the number of calories it takes your body to sustain life (normal metabolic functioning in a resting state). Another way to look at RMR is the number of calories it takes to sit around the house and do nothing all day long. This value equals about 70 percent of the total calories burned in one day. Exercise can indirectly affect your RMR because it takes more energy to sustain lean muscle mass than fat mass.
- In addition, the more fit you are, the greater the size and number of your mitochondria. Mitochondria are the little powerhouses in your muscles that burn calories. If you have more of them and they are bigger in size, your body is naturally burning more calories. Let's use another analogy. Think of mitochondria as furnaces: The more furnaces and the larger they are, the more fuel (calories) that can be burned.

Now let's combine the two analogies: (1) your body as a car and (2) your mitochondria as a furnace. The more you "run" your body, the more fuel, or calories, your body will expend and the more and bigger your mitochondria will become to facilitate the burning of more calories. As your body burns more calories, it decreases the size of its fat cells, resulting in weight loss. This phenomenon explains how exercise decreases fat by increasing the burning of fat. Your increased activity levels produce a better fat-burning body.

In addition, exercise, especially strength training, helps maintain or even increase your muscle mass. It takes more energy to sustain muscle or fat-free mass than fat mass; thus, additional calories are burned. As you decrease fat, maintain or even gain some lean muscle mass, and lose weight, you will ultimately lose inches because a pound of lean muscle is smaller in diameter than a pound of fat. This is also why you can lose inches but not always simultaneously lose weight.

HEALTH BENEFITS

In addition to its weight-loss benefits, exercise has a number of beneficial health effects. For those who want to increase their overall health or who are obese and have several other health problems, this is excellent news!

Regular exercise can improve overall cholesterol and can directly help increase high-density lipoprotein (HDL) and decrease low-density lipoprotein (LDL). HDL cholesterol is the healthy type; it helps break away plaque buildup in your arteries; LDL is bad because it contributes to buildup of plaque in your arteries. Exercise also lowers blood pressure, triglycerides, and blood sugar. For anyone who has high cholesterol, high blood pressure, or diabetes, exercise is the answer.

What about cancer? It seems everyone has at least one close friend or family member suffering from cancer? Why the increase in the incidence of cancer? Well, several studies have found a strong link between cancer and obesity. Experts estimate that in the United States, excess weight contributes to roughly [1]:

- One-half of all uterine and esophageal cancers.
- One-fifth (in women) to one-third (in men) of all colorectal cancers.
- One-third of all kidney cancers.
- One-quarter of all pancreatic cancers.
- More than one-fifth of all postmenopausal breast cancers.

I don't know about you, but this is alarming. I have a relative who has been suffering from stage IV ovarian cancer. When she was initially diagnosed, they gave her about three months to live. She fought through treacherous months of chemotherapy, radiation, and two radical surgeries and thought she was in remission only to find out about two months later that the cancer was back full force. Anyone you talk to who has been faced with the adversity of cancer will tell you that it's a very difficult road. For some, cancer is their final destiny. Start decreasing your cancer risk today by practicing healthy eating habits and exercising regularly. You can reduce your risk significantly if you keep your body mass index (BMI) at less than 25 or at a minimum under 30. See the following *New England Journal of Medicine* graphs depicting the relationship between extra weight and cancer risk in both men and women [2].

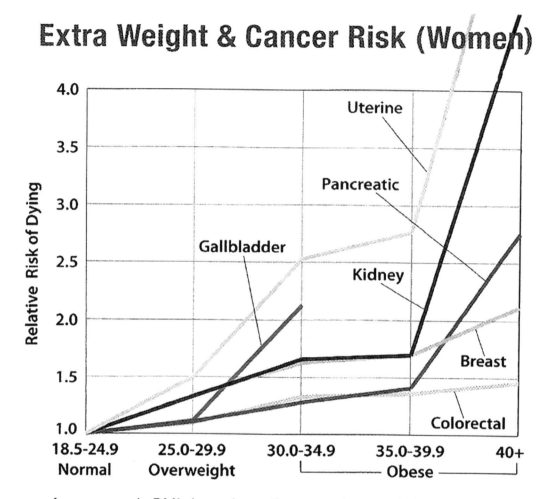

As a woman's BMI rises above the normal range (18.5 to 24.9), her risk of dying of several cancers also rises. For example, the risk of dying of uterine cancer is 50 percent higher for women who are overweight (a BMI between 25.0 and 29.9) than for women who are normal weight. For the most obese women (a BMI of 40 or higher), the risk is roughly six times higher. The line for gallbladder cancer stops early because there were too few deaths among the most obese women in this study to separate those with a BMI of 35 or greater.

Source: Data from New Engl. J. Med. 348: 1625, 2003.

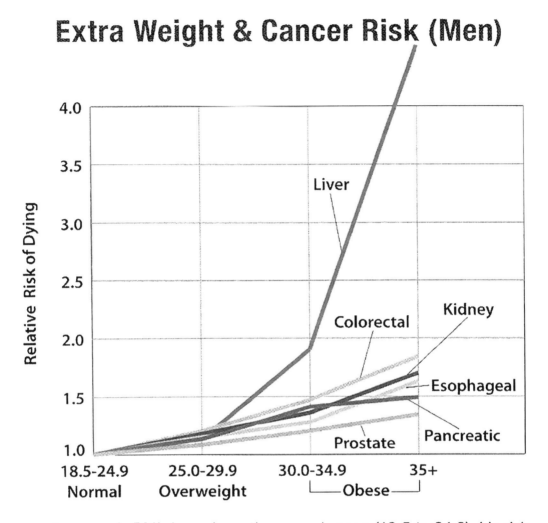

As a man's BMI rises above the normal range (18.5 to 24.9), his risk of dying of several cancers also rises. For example, the risk of dying of colorectal cancer is 20 percent higher for men who are overweight (a BMI between 25.0 and 29.9) than for men who are normal weight. For the most obese men (a BMI of 35 or higher), the risk is almost double (84 percent higher). This study had no separate data for men with BMIs of 40 or greater.

Source: Data from *New Engl. J. Med. 348*: 1625, 2003.

All of this information should begin to spark your motivation to become physically active. In addition to the previously mentioned health benefits, the following information should further motivate you:

- Regular exercise dramatically reduces anxiety, depression, and stress and lowers one's overall morbidity and mortality. Studies have suggested that between 112,000 and 365,000 premature deaths in the United States are due to obesity [3, 4]. It has been projected that extreme obesity shortens one's life span by 5 to 20 years [5, 6].
- A person's energy level, social life, and self-confidence are increased with regular exercise.
- Weight-bearing exercise helps improve bone and joint health, which in turn helps fight osteoporosis and arthritis.
- Exercise helps increase flexibility, strength, and cardiovascular fitness. These three improvements allow you to thoroughly *enjoy* your daily activities!
- As you grow older you may become weaker, overweight, fatigued, out-of-shape, have poor balance, bad posture, and the list goes on. Conversely, if you maintain or improve your physical fitness, which will help with long-term weight management, you will be able to fight or at least slow down the aging process and be able to do and enjoy most activities. Exercise is about the only fountain of youth you have, so take advantage of its benefits. Remember, if you don't use it, you'll lose it.

NOT "BUYING INTO" BUYING THE "MAGIC PILL"

If all of this exercise stuff could be packed into a magic pill, it would be much easier right? People have tried to do just that and they will continue to try. Just as I was beginning to write this book in February 2007, I heard a TV commercial about a new diet pill—the first non-prescription weight-loss drug approved by the FDA. The most telling thing about this new diet pill is that while the commercial touted the "benefits" of the pill, it stated that one must supplement the pill with a low-calorie diet and regular exercise.

It was alarming to me to hear this kind of press coverage about a weight-loss supplement. I couldn't believe they praised this pill on national TV, claiming it is the magic pill to help fight the obesity epidemic, but then essentially stated, "Oh, by the way, you will have to exercise and eat sensibly, too." The pill isn't helping you lose weight; it is the diet and exercise you do while on the medication. Oh, and you may experience gastrointestinal discomfort while taking the medication, according to the manufacturer. I will give this company the benefit of the doubt because it did not neglect to state that when taking the pill, you must also exercise in order to lose weight and combat obesity. However, I'm amazed to hear pitches about any "magic" pill or substance for weight loss. The truth is that you must simply increase your physical activity and modify your diet to reap weight-loss benefits. If exercise itself could be packed into a pill or other substance, it would probably be the most widely distributed product in the world!

I truly doubt there will ever be a pill that gives you all the benefits of exercise with no negative side effects. It is not good—in fact, unhealthy—to lose 10 lb in a month only to put 20 lb back on in three months. That is what happens when you go about dieting and exercising with the expectation of a quick fix. There really aren't any quick fixes, but I'm here to tell you that exercise doesn't have to be hard. Therefore, I urge everyone to stop looking for the "magic pill"! Stop looking for ways to get around exercise, and simply start exercising and maintaining a well-balanced diet. By doing this, you won't need a magic pill because you will reap more positive weight-loss and health benefits than any pill can provide.

GETTING MOTIVATED TO EXERCISE

Now you might be saying, "Yes, that sounds like a great idea, but I don't have any motivation to start moving. What can I do to get motivated?" Let's start with a detailed list of the specific benefits of exercise, an expansion of basic points about its benefits previously stated in this chapter. Exercise:

- Increases your daily caloric expenditure.
- Decreases body fat.
- Decreases inches.
- Increases or maintains fat-free body mass.
- Increases the body's fat-burning capacity.
- Improves cholesterol by decreasing LDL cholesterol and increasing HDL cholesterol.
- Lowers blood pressure.
- Lowers triglycerides.
- Lowers blood sugar and prevents or helps treat diabetes.
- Lowers risk for cancer.

- Reduces anxiety and depression.
- Relieves stress.
- Lowers mortality rate.
- Improves energy levels.
- Improves self-confidence.
- Improves social life.
- Strengthens bones and helps prevent osteoporosis.
- Improves flexibility.
- Improves cardiovascular health.
- Improves strength.
- Improves balance.
- Prevents falls.
- Improves ability to carry out daily activities.

Knowing now that regular exercise provides this many benefits, are you ready to start? Exercise is most important for long-term weight-loss success. Don't forget that the goal is not only to lose weight but also to keep it off for good. Maybe you have the best of intentions, but if every time you start exercising, you end up stopping, you are not maintaining consistency and thus losing ground. This is often the case for many people. It isn't that they can't find the motivation to start; it is *sticking with it* that is most difficult.

RECOGNIZING OBSTACLES

The first thing to do is recognize some of the obstacles that get in the way and prevent you from either getting started or sticking with your exercise program. Here are some of the classic reasons (excuses) I've heard throughout the years:

- I just don't have enough time.
- I'm too busy with my job, taking care of my family, taking care of housework (i.e., cleaning and/or yard work), or going to school.
- I don't really know what to do or how to get started.
- I'm too old to exercise.
- Every time I start, something comes up and I can't seem to follow through.
- I have so many physical limitations that I can't really exercise much, and when I do, it hurts.
- I don't have any motivation.

- I'm tired all the time.
- I hate exercise and, in general, I don't enjoy physical activity.
- I have a gym membership, but I don't feel comfortable going there.
- When I start to exercise, I often end up getting hurt and can't continue.
- Exercise is boring to me.
- I get enough exercise at work and home.
- I have too many health problems to exercise.
- I can't afford a gym membership.
- I don't have the right equipment at home.
- I hate to sweat.
- I care for little children and can't break away from them.

Do some of these reasons (rationalizations) sound familiar? I'm sure you can relate to some or most of these obstacles. Let's discuss ways to surmount them.

Remember, you must be ready to make a commitment to your own health and well-being. Are you serious about losing weight and improving your health? If so, you must be ready to work around your obstacles. If you don't feel like you are ready yet, do some more self-examination. Understand where you are today, where you want to be, and where you will be if you don't make some lifestyle changes.

OVERCOMING OBSTACLES

Since many of you can relate to the previously mentioned rationalizations, let's spend some time discussing how to work through each barrier.

I JUST DON'T HAVE ENOUGH TIME.

Time is probably the biggest obstacle, especially if you are trying to work full-time, care for your family, and accomplish household chores. Or maybe you are going to school on top of all these other daily responsibilities. It just seems like there is never enough time in the day. Since time is one of the biggest obstacles, it will be important for you to sit down and look at your weekly schedule. Determine what is getting in the way of your ability to find time to exercise. Are there any times during your day that aren't that productive; i.e., watching television, going out for lunch every day, or sleeping more hours than necessary. Can you cut some of this time down and replace it with exercise? Examine what times are best for your physical activity (e.g., mornings, afternoons, or evenings). Maybe, you can squeeze some exercise in during your lunch hour? Maybe, you can wake up 30 minutes early and do a workout before you go to work. How about right after work—can you stop at the gym to workout a couple days of the week? We all have different schedules, so you will have to determine what time is best for you.

I am often asked what time of the day is best to exercise. My response is always this, "I don't really care when you exercise as long as you exercise and you are consistent." There is a lot of controversy out there as to what time of the day is best. As long as you are exercising, you will reap the benefits. Spend more time determining what will work best for your schedule. That will determine what time of the day is best for you.

I'm too busy with my job, taking care of my family, and taking care of housework (i.e., cleaning and/ or yard work).

It is true that everyone is busy, but you have to make time to exercise. If your reason for not exercising is because you have to take care of your family, what happens when your health gets in the way of your ability to take care of your family? I have seen people get themselves into a position in which their health affects their ability to take care of their family and/or hold down a job. Believe it or not, you will have more energy if you exercise on a regular basis.

Put things in perspective. When I set people up on an initial exercise program, I'm usually only asking for two to four hours per week of that person's time. Considering there are seven days in a week, with 24 hours in each day, I don't think 2-4 hours is asking too much, especially if it means taking care of yourself so that you can take care of your family, job, and house. Don't forget that exercise has been proved to give you numerous health benefits as previously mentioned, so, if you keep yourself in shape, you will be able take care of all your responsibilities more easily.

Many companies are beginning to realize that improved health means less work missed and higher productivity while at work; thus, some companies offer different wellness benefits, such as a gym membership, free health screenings, or fitness program. An article in the *San Antonio Express News* suggests that obesity is affecting our economic health. In the article, Helen Darling, president of the National Business Group on Health states, "Obese workers on average, cost employers 56 percent more than employees in their ideal weight range" [7]. Due to this alarming statistic, many state and city officials are urging community and business leaders to make improving the health of the community's citizens a priority.

Treat your exercise time as *"sacred" time.* This is time for you! Make it as important as a doctor's appointment. Most of us wouldn't miss a doctor's appointment, so why let things get in the way of your exercise time? Besides, it is proven that spending more time exercising means less time at the doctor's office. Those who exercise regularly tend to get sick less often and have a better immune system.

In addition to finding time to exercise, begin to incorporate more and more activity in your daily lives. Do simple things like taking the stairs instead of the elevator, parking further away from buildings, walking to the mailbox, cleaning house, washing your own car, washing the dishes, standing instead of sitting, etc. All of these activities will burn extra calories each day. This will add up over time, resulting in a few extra pounds shed.

I DON'T REALLY KNOW WHAT TO DO OR HOW TO GET STARTED.

This rationalization underscores the reason I wrote this book. Hopefully, you are reading this book to understand how to exercise—specifically, how to exercise for weight loss. By the time you finish reading this book, you should have a pretty good understanding of how to get started with exercise and how to progress in order to maximize your weight loss. Of course, there is a lot more to learn about exercise. I always encourage my clients to seek a fitness professional for additional guidance. The key is to know what to look for in a fitness professional. I have outlined exactly what to look for in the last section of this chapter. Please refer to this chapter before hiring or seeking professional fitness counsel.

I'M TOO OLD TO EXERCISE.

This one "kills" me! You are never too old to exercise—much like you are never too old to stop learning. In fact, if you are aging, this is all the more reason to exercise. Remember, exercise is the only thing that slows down the aging process. In addition, exercising and increasing your strength and balance can help you avoid spending time in the hospital. Several older people end up in the hospital or nursing home because they fell and broke a hip or some other bone. The reason they fall is because they have poor balance and their muscles atrophy or become weak. By incorporating some light stretching and strength training, you can improve strength, balance, bone health, and posture. This in turn prevents falls and allows you to be independent.

EVERY TIME I START, SOMETHING COMES UP AND I CAN'T SEEM TO FOLLOW THROUGH.

This is a common rationalization. Everyone has good intentions, but it seems our efforts get derailed by some kind of distraction. You may start off real well and then get sick, or there is a death in the family, or your job becomes stressful. Some of these things cannot be helped. Life is full of surprises, so you have to anticipate disruptions. Remember to treat your exercise as sacred time. Do everything you can to prevent other things from taking precedence over the time you have set for you.

Of course, some disruptions will cause some setback in your physical activity (e.g., getting sick). Listen to your body. If it needs rest, give it rest. Just remember to get back on track after things settle down. It's okay to get off track for a while, provided you can get yourself back on track. And don't get frustrated if you can't always do your normal workout; maybe for a while you have time for only half of your workout, but this is better than no workout at all. If you do have to take a week or two off from your exercise regimen, remember to get back into it and start slowly. Don't expect to pick up right where you left off.

I have so many physical limitations that I can't really exercise, and when I do, it hurts to exercise.

For someone with physical limitations who is beginning to exercise, it is important to seek a fitness professional who knows how to work around the limitations. If you have physical limitations, a knowledgeable fitness instructor can help you overcome or, at least, work around those limitations. Let me give you an example.

I had a client who came to me with quite a bit of apprehension. This client was physically disabled from her job and was in pain about 80-90 percent of the time. Her biggest limitation was her back. She had disc fusions and a couple of herniated discs in her cervical and lumbar spine. She also had sciatica in her leg and had a torn rotator cuff. She was stricken with fibromyalgia and, consequently, her muscles ached most of the time.

Due to these complications, her body was in constant pain and she was fearful of injuring her back even more. She didn't know if she could exercise, and, if she did, she didn't know how to do it without injuring herself. I explained to her that exercise would provide relief for her conditions as long as she exercised the right way. I was excited about working with her and explained to her that I would have her start exercising slowly, first rehabilitating her back and shoulder, to help alleviate some of the pain she was experiencing.

I was looking forward to helping her feel better, and I was confident it would happen. I explained my qualifications, as I could tell she was still a bit nervous. She became convinced that exercise would help her and made an appointment with me. I told her exercising in a pool would be the best place for her to start because it would have a lower impact on her joints. So the pool is where we began. I started her in a therapeutic pool, which is warmer in temperature than a regular swimming pool. The temperature stays about 92 degrees Fahrenheit (F) and this warmth has a therapeutic effect on aching joints and muscles. This is important for individuals suffering from joint pain due to arthritis or from other mobility-limiting factors.

My main focus was to help her strengthen the muscles around the affected joints to alleviate pain and increase overall range of motion, allowing her to function more easily in life. Basically, I wanted her to strengthen the muscles around her joints so that the muscles would take on the bulk of the weight-bearing role rather than her joints.

As she progressed through training, she started feeling better. She stated several times that she always felt better when she came to do her pool exercises. On one occasion, she said the exercise felt better than a glass of wine or any other pleasure she enjoyed because the exercise took the pain away. She continued to progress in her pool exercises and ultimately transitioned to more land based activities. The physical training allowed her to enjoy daily activities and live a life that was much less painful than when she wasn't exercising on a regular basis.

This is one of many examples of how effective exercise can be, especially for those suffering several physical limitations. With appropriate exercise, many limitations can be overcome. I can't count the number of clients I have trained who originally came to me with severe knee and/or back pain and who are now pain free in those areas. Hopefully, this personal anecdote about a client's success will motivate you to overcome any physical limitation by seeking professional help and starting to incorporate activity that will help alleviate some of the pain and frustration associated with your limitation. Remember, exercise does not have to be painful.

I DON'T HAVE ANY MOTIVATION.

For most overweight or obese clients with whom I have worked, lack of motivation to exercise is probably one of their worst enemies. I hope some of the things you've read so far have sparked your motivation to exercise. If not, here are a few suggestions.

1. Seek a friend, family member, or co-worker to join you in your journey toward a healthier life.
2. If you can find someone to lean on for moral support and to help keep you accountable, you will tend to stay motivated to continue your journey. After all, you don't want to let the other person down.
3. If you can't find anyone to join you, you may want to start working with a personal trainer. Again, it is important to make sure he/she is qualified; however, personal trainers are great for increasing your motivation. This is what you are paying them for–to motivate you and help you to lose weight. They should coach you and cheer you on all the way. Your personal trainer will formulate an individualized exercise plan designed especially for you so that you can be successful and achieve your fitness goals. All you have to do is show up and be prepared to work. Even if you don't feel like working, that trainer will encourage you to push ahead and meet your weight-loss goals. When I, in a consultant capacity, see a client who is still struggling to find the motivation to exercise, I generally recommend he/she seek a personal trainer. Working with a personal trainer two to three times per week, or even one time per week, helps the person stay accountable to someone. Plus, the trainer can "mix it up" and keep workouts fun and entertaining. (See also the last section in this chapter.)

I'M TIRED ALL THE TIME.

If you are tired all the time, this is all the more reason to get moving. A sedentary lifestyle can contribute to fatigue; people who exercise on a regular basis have more energy and tend to have a better night's rest and get sick less often. You may think that exercise drains your energy, but ironically, it is quite the opposite. You may feel a little more fatigued the first few weeks, but once your body has adapted to exercising, you will have more energy than you ever had before.

I HATE EXERCISE–I DON'T ENJOY PHYSICAL ACTIVITY.

This statement is somewhat alarming to me because all of us have to be active in some form just to function in life. *Hate* is a pretty strong word. Most people who think they hate to exercise have this mind because they think they have to work really hard in order to lose weight. The old "no pain, no gain" mindset is long gone in today's fitness world. Exercise is really about getting your body moving, and it doesn't have to be boring. Look for activities that you enjoy so that exercise can be fun. How about swimming, playing tennis or golf, hiking, walking in the park, or walking in the mall? These are all forms of exercise that can be fun as well as help you become fit.

I HAVE A GYM MEMBERSHIP, BUT I DON'T FEEL COMFORTABLE GOING THERE.

This is common for many people. Identify an environment that *is* comfortable for you. Knowing what to look for in your exercise environment is key to feeling comfortable. An entire chapter is devoted to this topic; please refer to Chapter 3.

WHEN I START TO EXERCISE, I OFTEN END UP GETTING HURT AND CAN'T CONTINUE.

This obstacle goes hand-in-hand with the rationalization, "I have too many limitations to exercise." You must know what exercises are best for you, taking into account your fitness level, fitness goals, physical limitations, and other factors. Refer to Chapter 6 for specific exercise guidelines for particular limitations. You may also want to seek a fitness professional to understand how to exercise without injury.

EXERCISE BORES ME.

Exercise does not have to be boring. Spice it up a bit and try something new. Exercise with a friend, family member, or co-worker. Incorporate your physical activity into things you enjoy, such as hiking, golfing, gardening, other sporting activities, walking in the park, or some of the other fun activities mentioned above. There are thousands and thousands of exercises as well as different ways to set up an exercise program that will not be boring. Seek a fitness professional for ideas. Also, consider setting up your exercise environment in an area with entertainment such as a television, music, or video games.

I GET ENOUGH EXERCISE AT WORK AND HOME.

If your job or what you do on a daily basis at home keeps you physically active, then you are lucky. However, you will more than likely still need to incorporate at least two or three additional focused-exercise workout sessions into your weekly schedule. Even though you may be physically active at work, it probably isn't for an extended period of time. In other words, you may be active for a few minutes but then you usually have to stop to handle a situation before you resume physical activity, and this pattern continues throughout your work day. In order to reap the most benefits of cardiovascular exercise, you need to exercise for an extended period of time with little to no interruption. The same is true for strength training. Are you targeting every muscle group at work? Chances are slim that you will get a total body workout in the course of performing your job. This is why you should establish a more structured exercise regimen.

I HAVE TOO MANY HEALTH PROBLEMS TO EXERCISE.

Unless a doctor has specifically told you *not* to exercise due to a physical limitation or a medical condition, exercise will more than likely help the health condition(s) you have. Seek your doctor's advice. If your doctor says it is okay to start exercising, start moving. Be sure to exercise within the guidelines your physician gives. Again, in regard to exercise, you may want to seek a qualified fitness professional to help you work around a physical limitation or medical condition.

I CAN'T AFFORD A GYM MEMBERSHIP.

No problem. You don't need fancy equipment to get in shape. You can do several different exercises with your own body weight. In addition, you can take advantage of local parks for your fitness environment.

I DON'T HAVE THE RIGHT EQUIPMENT AT HOME.

Again, no problem. You can get in shape using your own body weight. In addition, you can purchase several inexpensive pieces of equipment for your home that will target the whole body. Resistance bands and stability balls are two examples of such equipment.

I HATE TO SWEAT.

Keep in mind that you don't have to work extremely hard to get in shape. This doesn't mean you won't sweat, but you probably won't sweat as much as you think. I'm not sure if I can tell you much more on this other than to wear fitness gear that helps wick away sweat (draws the sweat away from your body) to keep you dry.

I CARE FOR YOUNG CHILDREN AND CAN'T BREAK AWAY FROM THEM.

This is a classic obstacle for many people who have kids, especially if their children are still small and unable to care for themselves. There are several ways to work around this:

1. First of all, if you join a gym or are thinking about joining a gym, look for one that has a day-care center. That way, you can still workout while the gym's day care watches your kids.
2. If you don't join a gym and are planning on exercising at or near the home, see if your spouse, friend, neighbor, or even another family member is willing to watch your kids for a couple hours a week. That way, you can break away for some personal time and exercise at the same time. If this doesn't seem viable, try to arrange your workouts around your child's schedule.
3. If you are a stay-at-home mom or dad, try to get your workouts in while your kids are taking their daily nap.
4. Include your kids in your workout. There are several strollers on the market today that are built for walking moms and dads. Bring your kids along for the ride. You can even use your kids as resistance for some of your exercises. Remember the old airplane ride on mom or dad's feet. You can do this and then do some leg presses with your child in-between the airplane rides you give them. Picking your child up and down for several repetitions is also good exercise. Just make sure you are practicing proper lifting techniques. If your child is old enough, he/she can even do some of the exercises with you. Exercise can be a wonderful thing to do with the whole family.

Okay, no more excuses right? After discussing every obstacle you may face, the bottom line is that you have to make the commitment to be active. Remember, fitness is your key to long-term weight management. It is the only thing that significantly maintains or increases your metabolism. If you are losing weight through calorie restriction, this actually lowers your metabolism. The only way to combat this effect is to stay active.

So why are you waiting? Dedicate 20-30 minutes of your time, three or four times per week, to fitness. Start there and gradually progress. This only equates to 1-2 hours of your time in one week. I know you can make time for that, so be creative and find time. If you don't find the time now, you might have more time than you know what to do with later because you won't be able to do anything due to poor health. So, commit to exercising regularly and make a change today! For those of you who still cannot muster the necessary motivation and commitment, working with a fitness professional may be the key.

FINDING AND WORKING WITH A QUALIFIED FITNESS PROFESSIONAL

One of the best ways you can create a successful and innovative fitness program is to seek the assistance of a qualified fitness professional. Somebody who does this every day for a living can help you stay on track with your exercise program. He/she can also keep you accountable, help you progress with your exercise, make sure you don't get hurt, and ensure you don't get bored or hit a plateau and cease to make progress. The key is to make sure the professional you seek is well qualified. Unfortunately, the fitness industry has not set standardized credentials, education, and experience to differentiate good or excellent fitness instructors from mediocre or bad ones.

Today there are trainers teaching people how to exercise whose sole credential is a certification they received in one weekend or maybe on the Internet. This is not the kind of trainer you want to find. Now, I'm not saying that they are poor at doing their jobs, but your chances of finding someone who is well-versed in working with your medical conditions and/or restrictions, as well as meeting or surpassing your weight loss goals, are slim. So, how do you know if the fitness professional is good or not? Look for the following credentials in fitness professionals:

1. Undergraduate or higher degree in an exercise-related field (e.g., exercise science, exercise kinesiology, exercise physiology, health and wellness, physical education, or sports science
2. One or more nationally recognized fitness certifications from one of the following organizations:
    - American College of Sports Medicine
    - National Academy of Sports Medicine
    - American Council on Exercise
    - American Fitness Professionals & Associates
    - International Fitness Professionals Association
    - Cooper Institute
    - National Strength and Conditioning Association
3. Current CPR/AED certification through the American Heart Association
4. At least one or more years experience (Be sure to ask them what their specialty is, for example, bariatrics, geriatrics, pediatrics, sports medicine).

Also, to really see if your trainer/fitness professional knows his/her stuff, ask them one or two of these four questions:

1. *What does a beta blocker do to your heart rate?* Beta blockers are blood pressure medications designed to suppress the heart rate by blocking the hormone epinephrine, which results in dilating the blood vessels and causing the blood to flow easily through the vessels. Beta blockers are frequently prescribed by physicians for the following conditions: high blood pressure, irregular heart beat, heart failure, chest pain, heart attacks, glaucoma, migraines, anxiety disorder, hyperthyroidism, and certain types of tremors.
2. *Does the fitness professional have a complete health history questionnaire and/or Physical Activity Readiness Questionnaire (PAR-Q) before you start exercising?* Completion of the Physical Activity Readiness Questionnaire (PAR-Q) before starting an exercise routine flags a client who needs additional exercise clearance. It is an industry standard for a fitness professional to ensure that a client has completed a PAR-Q prior to directing exercise for the individual, unless the client has provided the fitness professional with written exercise clearance from a physician. Before a fitness professional starts you on an exercise program or allows you to work out in their gym or fitness center, she/he should take notes on your health history and ask you to complete a PAR-Q.
3. *If you have or develop a heart condition, does the fitness professional get additional clearance from your primary care physician (PCP) or cardiologist?* Obtaining clearance from your PCP or cardiologist is an industry standard. If you suffer from any type of heart condition, your fitness professional should receive clearance from your PCP or cardiologist before you start a comprehensive exercise program.
4. *What about weight loss? What is the best way for you to exercise if your primary objective is weight loss?* In order to be most successful with weight loss, your fitness professional should encourage both cardio and strength training, with more of a focus/emphasis on cardio because this is where you will burn the most calories (specifically, fat calories). Strength training is important so that you can maintain or even increase a little lean muscle through the weight-loss process. This helps to keep your metabolism up, which will help burn more total calories on a daily basis. Chapter 4, Understanding and Building on the Four Pillars of Fitness, and Chapter 7, Maximizing Your Body's Fat-Burning Capacity, give detailed information on exercising for weight loss.

These are just a few basic questions to ask a prospective trainer/fitness professional. A well-qualified one should know the answers. Once you have identified a fitness professional who is well educated, qualified, and experienced, have him/her modify your exercise program every four to six weeks. You should not stay on the exact same program longer than that. Remember that exercise is stress to your body. Once your body gets used to the stress, it adapts to it and plateaus—that is, it ceases to respond physiologically in a manner that contributes to weight loss and loss of inches. In order to maintain an appropriate amount of stress and keep your body and muscles "guessing," you must change your exercise routine on a regular basis (i.e., every four to six weeks). This is a form of periodization, which means breaking up one's training program into different phases to maximize specific training goals.

REFERENCES

1. Liebman, Bonnie. Cancer: how extra pounds boost your risk. *Nutrition Action Health Letter* 2007;34(7)(September):3.
2. Calle, E, Rodriguez, C, Walker-Thurmond, K, Thun, M. Extra weight & cancer risk (women & men). *New England Journal of Medicine* 2003;348:1625.
3. Flegal, KM, Graubard, BI, Williamson, DF, et al. Excess deaths associated with underweight, overweight, and obesity. *Journal of the American Medical Association* 2005;293 (15):1861-1867.
4. Mokad, AH, Marks, JS, Stroup, DF, et al. Actual causes of death in the United States. *Journal of the American Medical Association* 2005;293(3):293-294.
5. Fontaine, KR, Redden, DT, Wang, C, et al. Years of life lost due to obesity. *Journal of the American Medical Association* 2003;289(2):187-193.
6. Peeters, A, Barendregt, JJ, Willekens, F, et al. Obesity in adulthood and its consequences for life expectancy: a life-table analysis. *Annals of Internal Medicine* 2003;138:24-32.
7. Polin, Travis E. Is San Antonio's high rate of obesity scaring away business? *San Antonio Express News,* November 28, 2007.

Chapter 3
Creating Comfort in Your Fitness Regimen

In order to better understand a comfortable environment as it relates to fitness, it is important to define the words *environment* and *comfortable*. *Environment* can be defined as (1) the conditions, influences, and things that surround (2) all other external factors that affect an organism at any time, and (3) the social and cultural conditions that shape the life of a person or population [1]. Basically, this means you should find a place to exercise with the conditions, factors, material things, and social and cultural influences that allow you to feel comfortable. Knowing what to look for is half the battle.

So what exactly is "comfortable"? Too many of us think that a big bed with fluffy pillows is the most comfortable thing or place to be. I would agree that a bed is probably one of our most comfortable environments, but there are many places where you can feel comfortable. You just need to understand what to look for. The word *comfortable* is defined in the following ways: (1) providing physical comfort, (2) free from stress or anxiety, (3) a condition or feeling of ease, and (4) more than adequate or efficient [1].

If these two words (*comfortable* and *environment*) are combined into one definition as it relates to finding a comfortable fitness environment, the definition would be something like this: a place or surroundings that is more than adequate. In other words, it exceeds your expectations and surrounds you with external factors or conditions that produce a state of physical and mental ease or comfort.

Wow! That is where I want to be. Maybe you are not convinced yet. I'm not saying you will always feel comfortable when you exercise, but the environment in which you exercise should definitely provide some comfort. In order to be successful with your exercise routine, it is paramount that you're at ease while you exercise.

Hopefully, this environment will become so comfortable that you will not want to miss your exercise. If you do miss your exercise, you will miss the comfort the exercise environment provides. It is when you reach this comfort level that you know exercise is now part of your daily life. It's your lifestyle! If you miss your workouts you'll feel more sluggish, have less energy, and feel the need to get moving. This is when you've really accepted exercise as being part of your life. You might think this will never happen to you, but believe me, it can happen and it's a wonderful thing!

So how do you find a comfortable fitness environment? You should define the environment in which you plan to exercise, recognize what to look for in a fitness center, identify fitness equipment that works for you, be familiar with what to wear, and recognize appropriate qualifications when choosing a fitness staff to help you with your exercise.

The first thing you will need to identify is the type of environment in which you will be exercising. This depends largely on your schedule as well as your financial situation, exercise restrictions or limitations, and your weight loss and fitness goals. Let's take a good look at four common fitness environments: the home, park, "on the road" travel environment (e.g., hotel), office, or gym/fitness center. Most people exercise in one or more of these environments.

WORKOUT LOCATIONS (ENVIRONMENTS)

THE HOME

The home is a common environment for many people because it is convenient. You don't have to worry about hours of operation, other people using your machine, other people watching or looking at you, or packing your gym bag for the road. However, some people can't use their home as a primary fitness environment because there are too many distractions or there may not be as much variety when exercising in the home. This is why you have to define the environment that is best for you. It may be comfortable, but if it is not meeting your needs, you may want to consider changing your environment.

If the home is to be your primary fitness environment, you should consider several isues as you set up an exercise area in your home:

1. What time of day do you plan on exercising?
2. Where do you plan on exercising? Pick a place that is not going to disturb others or yourself.

3. Is the location big enough for all of the things you want to accomplish?
4. What type of equipment do you plan to use?

I've worked with people who have anything from a full gym in their house to nothing at all. Obviously, the more equipment you have, the more variety you will have; however, you can get a great workout with minimal equipment or no equipment at all. A mirror is an item that is good to have so that you can monitor proper form while executing your exercises. This is especially true for strength training. You will need to analyze whether or not the equipment you have allows your exercise routine to incorporate flexibility, cardiovascular, and strength training, while accommodating for any restrictions or limitations you may have. I discuss the four pillars of fitness as well as how to work around exercise restrictions and limitations in Chapters 4 and 6, respectively.

HOTELS

If you travel frequently for your job or for pleasure, you will more than likely use a hotel for your fitness environment. Many hotels have fitness centers in them or they have a contract set up with a local gym so that guests can use that gym's facility as long as they stay at the hotel. If neither one of those options are available, you can always pack a resistance band or stability ball and have a gym right in your room.

Many people use travel as an excuse for lack of physical activity, but that is just what it is—an excuse. Remember that once you have embraced a lifestyle change, you must work and plan ahead to fit physical activity into your daily routine. Make it a priority rather than something you'll get to when you have time. Trust me, you will never find time. If you believe you don't have time to exercise, re-read the first two chapters.

OFFICE

Depending on your employer, you may be fortunate enough to have a fitness center where you work. If this is the case, take advantage of this wellness benefit. Many people would love to have this opportunity and convenience to help them get fit and stay fit. Maybe you don't have a full gym, but you can certainly do three or four different office exercises each day that are beneficial for your flexibility and circulation and break up the monotony of the computer, telephone, and other sedentary work activities. For example, you can take 5-minute breaks every few hours and stretch, do basic chair exercises, walk down the hallway or around the office building, or just do some deep breathing. This will help relieve tension as well as produce circulatory and flexibility benefits. Other activities you can perform in the office during the course of your daily tasks include taking the stairs instead of the elevator, parking further away from your office building, walking to a co-worker's office instead of calling or using email, and planning and bringing a healthy lunch to work. If you routinely eat lunch out, you have less control over your dietary choices and risk eating larger portions, more processed, fatty, and high-sodium food.

PARKS AND TRAILS

Maybe you live close to a park or simply like to be outside when you exercise. If so, this may be your optimal exercise environment. You can get a great workout in a park if you know how to use your own body weight and different things available to you in the park. You may decide to bring a small piece of equipment with you. If the park is your primary exercise environment, always have a backup plan in case of inclement weather.

Things to look for in a park include trails, terrain, hours of operation, distance from home or office (proximity), and safety.

TRAILS, TERRAIN, AND HOURS OF OPERATION

If you are looking for a place to walk or jog, you need to know if the park has trails as well as the terrain of those trails. If the trails are unpaved, you will want to wear appropriate footwear for that terrain. Some parks have trails with different exercise stations built along the trail. This is a great feature to find in a park because it will help guide you through your workout.

PROXIMITY

Generally speaking, you will want to pick a park that is in close proximity to your home or office. Your commute to the park should optimally be 10-15 minutes. Most parks have fixed hours of operation, which often change with the season or daylight savings time. Check to see if these hours match the time of day you will be working out.

SAFETY

If you are a nighttime or early morning exerciser, make sure the park is well lit so that you can see where you are going and be alert to any unsafe situations that may arise. Speaking of safety, a park can be a dangerous place to exercise if you are not prepared. If your park has trails, make sure you review the trail map before you start. Establish a route that fits your fitness level. Keep your map with you at all times in case you get lost. If the trails are long and off road, take a first-aid kit in addition to a compass and/or global positioning system (GPS). Many GPS systems today are small and inexpensive. This is another way to make your workouts fun!

Carry a cell phone and always make sure you tell someone where you are going before you leave. It is also a good idea to carry a small can of mace in case you come across a threatening or aggressive person or animal. You should select a park that is located in a safe area of town and one that doesn't have any bad stigma associated with it. Simply watch the local news on the television or check the Internet to ensure the park you choose doesn't have crimes regularly occurring in it (e.g., drug bust, assault).

Last, make sure you bring plenty of water so that you can stay hydrated, and depending on the length of your walk or hike in the park, you may want to pack a healthy snack.

GYM OR FITNESS CENTER

Last but not least, maybe your ideal environment is a gym or a fitness center. There are several things to look for in a fitness-center environment.

PROXIMITY AND HOURS OF OPERATION

Like a park, your gym should be in close proximity to your home or office. There have been studies that show a commute greater than 12 minutes may hinder your commitment in going to the gym because it takes more time from your busy schedule [2]. Be sure the hours of operation are in line with the times you intend to workout.

CLEANLINESS

Cleanliness of the facility is also very important because you don't have time to get sick. According to Phillip Tierno, the Director of Microbiology at New York University Medical Center, 80 percent of all infectious diseases are transmitted by direct contact with an infected person or indirect contact (contact with an object an infected person has touched or, in the case of airborne infections, that an infected person has breathed on, or in the vicinity of) [3].

Initial appearances can tell you a lot about how the facility is being run. If the equipment is not clean, there is no telling what else might be wrong.

SAFETY

You should also evaluate the safety of the center. Make sure the fitness staff are CPR- and AED-certified (*CPR* stands for cardiopulmonary resuscitation, and *AED* stands for automated external defibrillator.). The American Heart Association has incorporated AED training into their CPR training because the combination of CPR and early defibrillation greatly increases a heart attack victim's chance of survival. So, check to see if the facility has a working AED.

Other important safety features to look for in a gym or fitness center are:

- Staff members who are available to help spot you during your workout.
- Mirrors positioned in free weight areas to ensure proper form.
- Well-maintained equipment.
- A floor that is free of tripping hazards.
- Aquatic or locker rooms with slip mats in the wet areas.

COST OF MEMBERSHIP AND SERVICES PROVIDED

The cost of membership is yet another thing to research in a fitness center. Don't be afraid to shop around: Do a cost comparison of the gyms you are considering. Be aware of hidden fees, such as contracts, start-up fees, etc. These things may lock you into an uncomfortable environment. Evaluate what each facility has to offer, such as ancillary services. Maybe you have kids and will need some type of child care during your workouts. What about nutritionist, mental health, or physician care? Wouldn't it be nice to have them all under one roof so that the different providers can work together to ensure you meet your weight loss goals? There is much more to weight loss than fitness, so it is nice to have other support staff at your disposal.

SIZE AND DEMOGRAPHICS OF MEMBERSHIP

The size and demographics of the gym may greatly affect your comfort level while exercising. Do you prefer a small or large facility? There are pluses and minuses to both. Do you feel intimidated by large facilities with tons of different fitness equipment? Maybe this makes everything more confusing because you just don't know where to start. Or, maybe you like more variety in your workouts, so the larger facility with several choices is best for you. Take the size of the facility into consideration along with the types of members the gym attracts. Does the gym cater to children, college students, body builders, athletes, or a geriatric population? A gym that specializes in bariatrics or weight loss would be ideal because, more than likely, the gym has been set up with this population in mind. People tend to feel most comfortable around members who are striving for similar goals, such as weight loss.

EQUIPMENT

The equipment in your fitness-center environment is very important. In fact, the equipment is probably one of the main reasons why you chose the gym as your primary environment. With this in mind, what do you need to look for in equipment to make sure you are able to effectively pursue your weight-loss exercise program?

First, determine if the equipment allows for easy entry and exit in relationship to your size. In other words, can you safely get on the equipment, begin to exercise without any restriction, finish exercising, and safely get off the equipment? If the answer is "yes," you have found the appropriate equipment.

Next, determine if the facility has enough equipment for you to perform all aspects of your fitness program: flexibility, cardio, and strength. Let's consider a scenario: You are a 5' 5" female who weighs 245 lb, and your limitations include severe arthritis in your knees, low back pain, and a right drop foot. A drop foot is a condition in which you're unable to bring the foot upward (i.e., dorsiflex). The foot involuntarily drops down or pronates (excessively rolls inward after the initial foot strike). Due to your excess weight and severe knee pain, the treadmill, bicycle, elliptical trainer, and stair stepper are not the best cardiovascular machines for you. You'll need a fitness center that has an upper extremity bike or aquatic program because these two forms of cardiovascular exercise are low impact on the joints, specifically the knees. They will allow you to safely and most effectively perform your cardiovascular exercise program. Similarly, you will want to look for strength equipment that does not put undue stress on your knees. Chapter 6 discusses in detail what you need to consider if you have a particular limitation or medical problem.

If you look at the different types of fitness equipment, visualize yourself getting in and out of the equipment. Will you be able to easily get in and out? Does the equipment make you feel comfortable? Are the seats of the various exercise machines big enough? Will the treadmills and stability balls support your weight? Are the towels big enough for your body? These are questions you'll want to answer and they are also things that shouldn't cause you anxiety while working out in your fitness center. The bottom line is that you need to identify equipment that is going to work for you and make you feel comfortable. Take a look around and start thinking about this before you lock yourself into a fitness-center membership.

If your environment is a home, office, or hotel, try to find equipment that is compact and easy to transport, such as resistance bands, stability balls, small hand weights, a body bar, or your own body. You can build a good total body strength routine with any or all of these pieces of equipment.

The resistance band is probably the most versatile and easiest piece of equipment to transport next to your own body. Of course, you can use a good pair of shoes and your own body to create an excellent cardiovascular piece of equipment. Simply walking, jogging, or running produces a great cardio workout. What if you have severe knee pain? Well, walking or jogging is not going to be a viable option. If this is the case, you will need to seek another option such as a pool or an upright or recumbent bike—some exercise that will not create a lot of stress on your joints is good. It is very important to identify your restrictions and understand what exercises to avoid when identifying your fitness environment. Pick an environment that allows you to do all of your exercises without jeopardizing your limitations and causing an injury.

WORKOUT ATTIRE AND GEAR

Once you have found a comfortable place to exercise, you need to consider what workout attire and gear you'll need. These are very important for feeling comfortable while you exercise. Have you ever gone out with your friends and felt miserable the whole night because your pants were too tight or you just weren't feeling good in your outfit? I know I have. Being uncomfortable in your clothes or shoes isn't fun. So what should you wear and take "to the dance"? If you want to maximize your comfort and overall attitude while exercising, you need to put some thought into the following three categories of workout attire and gear: (1) workout clothing, including shirts, shorts, pants, and undergarments, (2) athletic footwear, including shoes, primarily tennis shoes, and (3) workout accessories, including heart rate monitors, watches, water bottles, and sunglasses. See also Appendix A, Recommendations for Workout Apparel, Accessories, and Equipment.

WORKOUT CLOTHING

First and foremost, your exercise clothing should be loose fitting to allow for a full range of motion while exercising. Wear clothes that don't restrict you from movement while performing your exercise. In addition, the type of clothing you choose should match your environment. For example, if you are exercising in the park in the fall or winter, wear clothing that is going to keep you warm (e.g., long shirt, sweat pants, jacket, gloves, hat). If your exercise environment is outdoors, dress in layers and be prepared for different types of weather.

Much of the athletic clothing today is made of a wicking-type material, which allows sweat to be wicked away from your body and keeps you comfortable while you perform your workout. This wicking feature keeps you warm in the cold and cool in the heat because the sweat does not stick to your skin. Sweat sticking to your skin can prevent your body's natural cooling/warming mechanisms from performing properly.

You can find all types of exercise clothes, from undergarments to shirts and pants, with this type of wicking material in them. So how do you know if your clothing has this wicking feature? Look for clothing that contains materials such as microfiber, Supplex, Lycra, polyester, Coolmax, nylon, or spandex. If you wear t-shirts that are 100-percent cotton, they may keep you damp and moist during most of your workout. Cotton is great for absorbing sweat but doesn't exactly dry quickly. If you look for clothing with a mix of one or more of the materials listed above, the clothing should keep you comfortable and dry for most of your workout.

ATHLETIC FOOTWEAR

Your shoes are yet another important piece of fitness gear. I cannot emphasize the importance of wearing appropriate footwear while exercising. I repeatedly see people exercise in shoes that are far from supportive, considering the activity in which they are engaged. Your feet take most of the load while exercising; thus, you should make sure your shoes can handle the load. This is even more important for overweight or obese individuals because their feet have to withstand a greater load on a continuous basis. If one's feet are not appropriately supported, the knees, hips, ankles, and/or back may carry the additional stress.

So how do you decide what type of shoes to wear? The first step is to make sure you look for *athletic/tennis* shoes to wear while exercising; there are several different kinds of athletic shoes to choose from. The second step is to identify the foot type you have. People generally fall into three different foot types: flat, normal arch, and high arch. The best way to determine the type of feet you have is to do what is called *the wet test*. Simply dip a bare foot into a bucket of water and then step onto a sidewalk or driveway. Identify the shape of your footprint and compare it to the chart below. Whatever footprint print looks closest to yours is the type of foot you have.

| Flat | Normal/Average Arch | High Arched |

Now that you know what foot type you have, you can find the appropriate shoe:

- *Flat:* If your feet are flat, look for motion-control shoes. Essentially, you want a shoe that reduces the degree of pronation in the foot. If you have flat feet, you already have a wide surface area that strikes the ground; therefore, you really don't want shoes that cause more motion of the foot, because you naturally have a lot of motion. Look for shoes with firm mid-soles and stay away from high-cushioned shoes or shoes that lack stability and control.
- *Normal/average arch:* If your foot has a normal or average arch, look for shoes with moderate-control features. In other words, your shoes should have some cushioning, support, and control and should allow for some additional motion to help guide the foot through each step.
- *High arch:* If you have a high-arch foot type, find shoes that are cushioned and offer plenty of flexibility to encourage foot motion. Unlike the flat foot, the high-arch foot does not have a large surface area that strikes the ground. Therefore, there is less movement/motion in the step and more stress on each part of the foot striking the ground. This is why it is better for people with high-arch feet to wear shoes that facilitate foot motion and provide additional cushioning to absorb the shock with each step.

This information on foot type will help you find the most comfortable exercise shoes. In addition to knowing the type of foot you have, you should also find a shoe that matches the majority of your activity. There are shoes that are best for walking, running, cross training, trail running/walking, basketball, softball, golf, and the list goes on. The next time you go to a shoe store, tell the sales person what type of foot you have and what type of activity you will be doing. This should help them match you with the perfect shoe.

It's almost time to start breaking in those new shoes, but first, let's consider some of the accessories that may complement your shoes and clothing.

WORKOUT ACCESSORIES

As for accessories, there are so many things to think about when deciding what to wear during your workout. Just keep in mind that you need to create the highest comfort level possible. If you know all the options, you will do a better job finding comfortable as well as practical accessories. There are many things to consider when accessorizing your workout wardrobe, so the following is a short list of accessories with a brief description of what to consider.

- *Heart rate monitors*: Find a monitor that allows you to program individualized heart rate training zones. Look for a monitor that gives you a reading of your average heart rate at the end of your workout and a total workout time. If you plan to exercise at dawn or dusk, you may want a heart rate monitor that offers a backlight so that the screen is illuminated in the dark. Many monitors give you readings on total calories burned and even tell you how much fat versus carbohydrates you've burned. This isn't a bad feature, but the values are often very inaccurate, since most monitors use demographic information (e.g., age, gender, weight) to calculate the values. One final feature is to find a monitor that is waterproof or water resistant, especially if you plan to use this in the pool or water.
- *Sunglasses*: Look for sunglasses with 100 percent UVA and UVB protection. Always wear protective eyewear when exercising outside, especially in full sun and/or snow. Sunglasses that are lightweight will be more comfortable.
- *Radios/MP3s/iPods*: Music tends to pass the time while exercising. There are so many different styles from which you can choose in this category, but if you don't have access to a computer, there is no need to buy an MP3 or iPod player. These devices require music to be downloaded from a computer. Please note that recent research has suggested that iPods can potentially affect a person's pacemaker. If you have a pacemaker and use an iPod, be sure to keep

the iPod a moderate distance from your heart. In other words, do not place it in your chest pocket or strap it around your upper arm.
- *Multimedia*: Whether it's music, a television, video games, a good book, or a fitness video, exercise is much more enjoyable with some form of multimedia. This can make a big difference in your comfort level and also helps pass the time while you exercise. Use exercise as a relaxation period, not another thing that adds stress to your life.
- *Hats/visors*: Hats and visors are options for protecting yourself from the sun's harmful rays. I recommend choosing hats and/or visors that are lightweight.
- *Waterbottles and/or Camelbacks*: Hydration is extremely important while exercising. If you do not have a water fountain or water that is easy to access while exercising, you should carry a water bottle with you. Camelbacks are great for hikes or long walks/runs. They are filled with water and simply rest on your back (like a backpack) while you exercise.
- *Watches*: During exercise, it is important to be aware of the time. It's also fun to monitor how long you've been exercising. The type of training you intend to do will determine the type of watch to buy. If you are training for some type of race (e.g., a 5K, 10K, half marathon, marathon, or triathalon), you may want to consider getting a watch that tracks lap times and/or interval splits. Similarly to the heart rate monitor, get a watch that is waterproof or water resistant, especially if you plan on wearing it in a pool or in wet weather. If you use a heart rate monitor, you may not need a separate watch, since most heart rate monitors have a watch built into them.
- *Compression wraps*: If you have an injury or joint that needs additional stabilization or support, a compression wrap may be your answer. I have one word of caution about compression wraps: Try to rehabilitate the area so that you don't have to depend on the wrap for long-term use. It may be an excellent accessory for short-term relief, but if you depend on it, you may make your injury or joint weakness worse because the muscles continue to "depend on" the compression wrap instead of becoming sufficiently strengthened to eliminate the need for the wrap.

TAKE-AWAY POINTS ON EXERCISE COMFORT

To recap the steps in identifying a fitness environment that you, personally, find comfortable:

1. First, determine your workout environment.
2. Next, identify the type of equipment you will be using while also considering your different limitations and restrictions.
3. Finally, choose appropriate fitness attire and accessories to provide the most comfort for your planned exercise activities.

In short, your exercise should be a comfortable experience. Don't just find an exercise environment—*create* your own total environment for maximum comfort. When you have accomplished this, you will be ready to begin your journey toward your wellness and weight-loss goals.

REFERENCES

1. Mokad, AH, Marks, JS, Stroup, DF, et al. Actual causes of death in the United States. *Journal of the American Medical Association* 2005;293(3):293-294.
2. McCullough, P, Gallegher, M, DeJong, A, et al. Cardiorespiratory fitness and short-term complications after bariatric surgery. *CHEST* 2006;(August)130:517-525.
3. Presidential Advice: Shake Off a Cold. Available at: www.medicinenet.com/script/main/art.asp?articlekey=50382.

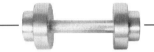

Part II

INITIATING AND MAINTAINING AN EXERCISE PROGRAM

Chapter 4
Understanding and Building on the Four Pillars of Fitness

From time to time, many of us have probably attempted to exercise in an effort to lose weight. The problem is that many of us exercise the same way we shop for groceries. When we go to the store, we often pick up the same items over and over again. We get used to certain foods and never venture out to incorporate more variety into our diets. This also is often the case with our attempts to become fit. Maybe you have said to yourself in the past, "I just don't understand why I can't lose any weight. I exercise five days a week and just can't seem to lose the weight. The only thing I lose is five days." As a fitness professional, my first question to you is "What exactly are you doing for your exercise?" You come back with, "Well, I walk for 30-45 minutes five times a week." And my next question is "Do you exercise at the same intensity all five days, and are you doing anything else besides walking?" Usually the response is, "Yes, I walk at roughly the same intensity, and walking is the only exercise I'm doing." Ah ha! Now I completely understand why you are struggling to lose weight."

Let me explain. First off, your exercise program is not well balanced. Much like your shopping regiment at the grocery store, you are choosing the same type of exercise over and over again, and you simply need more variety in your life. In addition, you are utilizing only one of the four pillars of fitness. Your body is smarter than that. You have to mix it up and make sure your exercise routine is balanced on all four pillars of fitness, which include flexibility, cardiovascular exercise, strength training, and a healthy, well-balanced diet. Think of these pillars as the four legs of a table. In order for the table to be sturdy and support what is placed on it, all four legs are necessary and they all need to be the same length.

If you took away one of the legs, the table would collapse. Similar to the table, your fitness program needs to incorporate all four pillars of fitness. Let's define each one of the four pillars and learn how to incorporate each one into your fitness program in order to maximize your weight loss and "keep your table from falling over!" First, let's consider the three pillars of fitness through exercise and then the fourth pillar, healthy dietary habits.

FLEXIBILITY (STRETCHING) EXERCISES

Flexibility, the first pillar of fitness, is simply the ability to move a joint through its complete range of motion. This is important because if you have poor flexibility, you will not be able to exercise to your full capacity or perform daily activities with ease. If you can improve your flexibility, you've facilitated movement in your joints, making it easier to accomplish daily activities.

So, when should you perform flexibility or stretching exercises? Many people think you should stretch before and after your workout. Actually, this is somewhat of a misconception: It is important to stretch only after the muscles have been warmed up; therefore, you should spend more time stretching after your workout. Stretching before your workout is okay, but you should warm up first, then do some light stretching, and then begin your workout. Or you can simply skip the stretching before working out and spend more time warming up before your workout. Appropriate warm-up exercises include walking or doing light cardio or calisthenics (e.g., walking, marching in place, or arm circles) at a lower intensity than you actually plan on doing for the duration of your workout. Warm-up exercises help increase blood flow, which will prepare the muscles for more advanced, strenuous movements. Stretching doesn't necessarily do much for increasing your blood flow, which is very important in order to get the oxygen and nutrients to the cells that need it during your exercise workouts. In short, it is best to stretch after your work out because then your muscles will be warmed up and you will get a better stretch, with lower risk for pulling a muscle.

Why is it important to stretch? Do you really benefit from stretching? You sure do! Let me explain. As mentioned above, flexibility is simply defined as the ability to move a joint through its complete range of motion. If you're not able to move a joint through its entire range of motion, that particular joint has somewhat of a limitation. In other words, you may not be able to do certain things with the muscles involved in the movement of a specific joint. This is problematic because most things we do in life require multi-directional movement across several joints.

Regular stretching provides three primary benefits:

1. Decreases the risk for injury during exercise and decreases muscle soreness after exercise.
2. Maintains the integrity of the muscle and prevents muscle imbalances, which can lead to poor posture. Essentially, stretching helps keep your muscles long, thus promoting good posture so that your muscles aren't pulling on different areas, causing tension and discomfort.
3. Decreases pain associated with arthritis, fibromyalgia, or other muscle and joint limitations.

There are three main factors to keep in mind while performing your flexibility exercises.

1. Stretching should never be painful.
2. You should stretch daily and hold your stretches for at least 10-30 seconds.
3. Do not bounce while stretching; hold a static or stationary position. This style of stretching is best for beginners.

What about yoga? Is it good for one's flexibility? Absolutely! In fact, yoga promotes both an increase in flexibility and muscular strength. Keep in mind that you can become too flexible. If your flexibility is beginning to jeopardize the stability of your joints, you may need to back off on your flexibility exercises. In other words, don't stretch or do yoga to a point at which you become "Gumby." Few people go to this unhealthy extreme in their stretching, but I raise the point to forewarn those who may mistakenly believe that more is better when it comes to exercise, particularly stretching exercises.

CARDIO EXERCISE

Cardiovascular/cardiorespiratory exercise—or cardio, as it is commonly known—is the second pillar of fitness. It is the activity of moving large muscle groups in a rhythmic motion for an extended period of time. This pillar of fitness is extremely important for weight loss because it increases caloric expenditure and improves your heart health. Exercises such as walking, biking, swimming, aqua jogging/walking, use of an elliptical trainer, rowing, arm cycling, stair stepping, rollerblading, skiing, and jogging are all cardio exercises.

Cardio exercise is critical for maximizing your body's fat-burning capacity during physical activity. All forms of exercise increase your ability to burn calories, but when you perform cardio exercise (also called aerobics or aerobic exercise), you burn more fat calories. Understand that your body utilizes two primary fuel sources while exercising: fat and carbohydrates. Protein is not an efficient fuel source. Some people think it is, but protein is really used to rebuild muscle tissue. Your body will generally tap into protein only during periods of extreme starvation. During aerobic exercise, your body utilizes oxygen. This is critical for burning fat; in fact, your body cannot metabolize fat without oxygen. This is why we tend to burn fat better at low to moderate levels of exercise intensity. In addition, it takes a lot longer to break down and metabolize fat versus carbohydrates due to the long-chain fatty acids that make up fat molecules. As you increase your intensity level, your body will need energy quicker. As a result, your system resorts to utilizing more and more carbohydrate for its fuel because it can get to it more quickly and break it down faster. This brings us to a discussion of glycogen.

We all have stored carbohydrates called glycogen that is readily available in our muscles. Exercising at higher exercise intensities forces the body to tap into its supply of glycogen to fuel it. It is important to note that exercising at higher intensities burns more calories per minute and helps increase the strength of one's heart. However, keep in mind that most people are not able to sustain long periods of high-intensity exercise; therefore, a greater total caloric burn can be achieved better at lower exercise intensities because one can exercise for longer periods of time. (This is especially true for unfit and overweight-to-obese individuals.) In addition, the body burns more fat during low-intensity exercise, and a lower intensity is "friendlier" to your joints, helping prevent injuries.

The main objective of your cardiovascular exercise should be to maximize your body's ability to burn fat. How to accomplish this is explained in detail in Chapter 7.

STRENGTH (RESISTANCE) TRAINING

Strength, or resistance, training—the third pillar of fitness—relates to the ability of the muscles to produce force or exertion. Resistance training involves a combination of improving muscular strength and muscle size, increasing one's muscular endurance, and maintaining lean muscle mass. The main objective of strength training for someone trying to lose weight is to maintain one's lean muscle mass through the weight-loss phase. This can be best accomplished through multiple strength-training sets and repetitions (i.e., 2-4 sets of 10-20 reps), which improves muscular endurance. If you can maintain your lean muscle mass through the weight-loss phase, you'll have a better chance of sustaining or even improving your metabolism. This is critical in sustaining a high level of caloric expenditure throughout the day. Understand that as you introduce a significant caloric restriction to the body, the body can tend to tap into one's lean muscle mass to make up for the calories lost. If you can supplement your diet with more protein, specifically lean protein, and begin to incorporate strength training you can minimize this loss of lean muscle tissue. Strength training will foster maintenance of, or even an increase in, lean muscle mass. This is important because one's lean muscle mass helps support a higher resting metabolic rate and overall metabolism. Strength training also promotes improved bone density, which helps prevent osteoporosis and improves the strength of muscles, ligaments, and tendons and thus directly impacts activities of daily living and reduces the risk of injury.

Now that three of the four pillars of fitness have been addressed, let's turn to the fourth pillar of *total* fitness, a healthy diet. It is important to incorporate all four pillars into your life to achieve and maintain your weight-loss goals and optimal health. Proper exercise and a healthy diet are inextricably tied together and must complement one another in a total fitness program.

HEALTHY DIET

You'll be happy to know that eating plays an integral part in becoming fit and healthy and that you don't have to "starve" yourself, skip meals, or go on some kind of major crash diet to lose weight. The answer to losing weight through diet is to choose the right kind of foods, keep your portion size in check, and ultimately burn more calories than you take in. To do the last of these, you must create a calorie deficit, but this doesn't mean you can't enjoy food. Creating a calorie deficit is not a daunting task if you know what your resting metabolic rate (RMR) is—that is, how many calories your body burns in one day to sustain itself in a resting state. One of the most accurate yet feasible and affordable ways to determine your RMR is through indirect calorimetry testing, also known as metabolic testing. If you know your RMR, then you'll know exactly how many calories to consume to lose weight. Keep in mind that there are 3,500 calories in 1 lb of fat, so if you create a 500-calorie deficit per day, you'll lose 1 lb a week (7 days in a week X 500 calories a day = 3,5000 calories, or a weight loss of 1 lb a week).

So what kind of food do you need to eat in order to lose weight and maximize your health? Let's start with the four macronutrients all foods contain: carbohydrates, fat, protein, and water. Then we'll briefly review how the consumption of alcohol may cause havoc in efforts to lose weight as well as cover the basics of vitamin and mineral recommendations. Special considerations for the weight-loss surgery patient will also be outlined. We'll wrap up with a sample weight-loss diet you can follow.

CARBOHYDRATES

Currently, the general population is still in a bit of the "low carb/no carb" diet craze, which really started when Dr. Atkins' came out with his *Atkins Diet*. I'm a firm believer in keeping the intake of carbohydrates (carbs) relatively low, but I definitely do not agree that carbs should be eliminated entirely. In fact, if you completely eliminate carbs from your diet, you'll feel very lethargic, since they are the body's main fuel source. In fact, glycogen (metabolized carbohydrates stored in the muscles and liver) is essential in order for muscle function (movement). If your main goal is weight loss, keep your carb intake at 40 percent or lower. In other words, 40 percent or less of the total calories you consume in one day should consist of carbs. By keeping your carb intake at 40 percent or lower, you'll force your body to tap into its fat stores and use fat rather than carbs as its fuel for energy. A sample diet consisting of 40 percent carbs is given at the end of this chapter.

Now, don't eat just any old carbohydrates. There are good (complex) carbs and not-so-good (simple) carbs. The good, complex carbs will not cause a spike in your blood glucose level; they require more calories to digest (break down); and consumption of them, specifically the consumption of dietary fiber, has numerous health benefits. It is recommended that you pair the complex carbohydrate foods you eat with a protein source in order to better stabilize your blood glucose levels. Make sure that 30-35 percent of the total 40 percent carbs you ingest consist of complex and dietary fiber carbohydrates; the other 5-10 percent can be simple carbs. Starches such as whole grain bread, sweet potatoes, corn, oatmeal, brown rice, green leafy vegetables, or whole wheat pasta are complex carbohydrates. Although food labels don't literally spell out "complex carbohydrate" or "simple carbohydrate," learn to read the label and understand whether or not the carbohydrate in a food is complex or simple. For example, if the first ingredient is whole grain, chances are that it's a complex carbohydrate. If one of the first ingredients is referred to as "enriched" or something similar, stay away from this particular food item, since all of the good stuff has been taken out through the processing of the food.

Studies have shown that diets rich in dietary fiber lower mortality rate, decrease the risk of heart disease and stroke, lower the risk of obesity, and decrease the risk of various forms of cancer [1]. Fiber also enhances satiety (sense of fullness and satisfaction) because when they are ingested, the emptying of the stomach occurs more slowly and glucose absorption does not happen as quickly. The National Cancer Institute recommends that an individual consume 20-35 grams (gm) of fiber each day [1]. Unfortunately, the average person falls far short of this recommendation. Foods that are high in dietary fiber include vegetables, fruits, beans, whole wheat breads, bran cereal, raisins and nuts. A unique feature of fiber is that some are completely insoluble, meaning that they pass through the entire gastrointestinal track unmetabolized, i.e., not broken down for absorption into the bloodstream, and thus act as a "free" carb since they don't account for a significant amount of calories. Additionally, insoluble fiber promotes regular bowel movements (preventing constipation), removes toxic waste, helps prevent colon cancer, and helps keep the pH optimal in the intestine. Green beans, green leafy vegetables, fruit skins, whole-wheat products, and nuts are all food sources that contain insoluble fiber. The soluble types of fiber also have beneficial metabolic effects, mainly decreased total cholesterol and blood sugar control (especially in diabetics).

Simple carbohydrates should be consumed in small amounts, especially if your main objective is weight loss. Simple carbs are basically comprised of glucose (sugar) and will add excess calories, cause a spike in your blood glucose, and subsequently lead to weight gain if they are not quickly utilized by the body for intense bursts of energy. If you do consume simple carbohydrates, choose their most natural state such as fruit (glucose or fructose) or milk (galactose or lactose).

FAT

Thank goodness the no-fat fad diets are not as prevalent as they were in the 1980s; however, fat as a macronutrient continues to get a bad rap. It is important to understand that fat is an essential nutrient and should not be completely eliminated from your diet; avoiding fat is no guarantee that you won't gain body fat. Consumption of some fat is necessary for proper cellular function, sufficient energy during aerobic exercise, transportation of fat-soluble vitamins to the various parts of the body through the bloodstream, and enhancement of satiety, or fullness, after meals. Try to keep your fat intake at 30 percent or lower; in other words, 30 percent or lower of the total calories you consume should consist of fat.

It is very important to be aware of the types of fat you consume. Similar to carbohydrates, there are good fats and bad fats. Monounsaturated and polyunsaturated fats are "heart healthy" because they help reduce cholesterol. Saturated and unsaturated (trans) fats are not heart healthy because they significantly increase overall cholesterol and ultimately increase the risk for heart disease. Always check food labels to see what kind and how much fat is contained in the product. Some examples of foods containing good fat include avocados, nuts, soy beans, fish, and vegetable oils. If you are trying to lose weight, the majority of your fat intake should be through consumption of lean meat and dairy servings, which also provide you with protein.

PROTEIN

Protein is not a major energy source for the body, but it is needed to build and repair body tissue. It forms the structural basis for muscle and synthesizes enzymes and hormones. For weight loss a moderate amount of lean protein in the diet, approximately 30 percent, is ideal to help preserve the lean muscle mass through the weight-loss phase. The idea is to force the body to burn fat both through diet and exercise. If you don't take in enough protein, you may actually break down your lean muscle mass and lose some of it through the weight-loss phase. You don't want this to happen because your lean muscle mass actually helps keep your metabolism up. You see, it takes more calories to sustain lean muscle versus fat, so you'll want to retain or even moderately increase your lean muscle in order to keep your metabolism up—"keep your furnace stoked," as some like to refer to it. The more lean muscle you have, the more calories your body will burn. This underscores the importance of strength training: Strength training will help maintain or even build lean muscle mass.

WATER

The body consists of about 50-60 percent water, which serves several functions. Water (1) carries nutrients and oxygen through blood to the cells that need it, (2) protects organs and tissue in the body, (3) lubricates joints, (4) regulates body temperature, and (5) helps dissolve nutrients and minerals so that the body can absorb them. Thus, it is very important to hydrate and continually replenish the body with water. Between 64 and 80 fluid ounces of water (eight to ten 8-ounce glasses) a day are recommended for most individuals. If you're more active, you'll need more water. For example, when you're exercising, you should drink half to one full cup of water (i.e., approximately four to eight swigs from a water fountain) every 15 minutes. Do not wait until you are thirsty; by then, you'll be on your way to dehydration. Limit caffeinated beverages, since they act as a diuretic contributing to fluid loss. As for sports or energy drinks, you generally do not need to drink either unless you're exercising for more than an hour. In these instances, you may want to use a sports drink to refuel, but keep in mind that you'll only need approximately 50-100 calories of carbohydrate every 45-60 minutes of exercise (this is only if you intend to continue exercising for more than an hour). The exact amount depends on the duration of your exercise session.

ALCOHOL

Alcohol per se (specifically ethyl alcohol) is not a food group but nonetheless contains calories; thus, its consumption can result in weight gain. In fact, alcohol contains quite a few calories in comparison to carbohydrate and protein; there are 7 calories per gram of alcohol versus 4 calories per gram of carbohydrate or protein—not to mention that alcohol is generally mixed with carbohydrates (e.g., margaritas, daiquiris, gin and tonic), which contributes to excess calories in every drink. In addition, it is important to understand that like fat, alcohol is metabolized in the liver. The liver essentially helps convert the metabolic by-products of alcohol into fatty acids. In short, alcohol is not the best thing to consume if your main objective is weight loss. Its consumption will essentially add excess calories to your daily caloric intake, which may ultimately be converted to body fat.

However, many people enjoy having a drink or two from time to time; therefore, it is important to talk about how much alcohol is recommended if you choose to partake. As with the consumption of any food or drink, drink alcohol only in moderation. One alcoholic drink is the equivalent of one 12-ounce bottle of beer, one 4-ounce glass of wine, or 1.25 ounces of liquor [1]. Thus, for the average male or female adult, drinking in moderation consists in having no more than one to two drinks daily. There are some studies that show light to moderate alcohol consumption reduces the risk of coronary heart disease and stroke.

The exact reason is unknown, but some suggest that small amounts of alcohol induce a relaxation effect, which reduces emotional stress (a risk factor associated with heart disease). Another theory suggests that light to moderate consumption of alcohol raises the level of HDL, the healthy form of cholesterol that helps protect against heart disease. Heavy drinking (three to six or more drinks a day) on the other hand, has shown to have adverse effects on one's health, including increased blood pressure, increased levels of blood lipids, increased risk for addiction or alcoholism, increased risk of pharyngeal and esophageal cancer, increased risk of cirrhosis (liver disease), mental impairment, increased risk of breast cancer, and increased risk of weight gain or obesity [1].

VITAMINS AND MINERALS

Vitamins are complex nutrients that aid in several functions of the human body. There are 13 vitamins: Nine (B_1, B_2, niacin, B_6, B_{12}, folic acid, biotin, pantothenic acid, and C) are water soluble, and four (D, A, K, and E) are fat soluble. Some vitamins are produced by the body, but most must be obtained from the food we eat. Due to this reason alone, depending on your dietary intake, your health care professional may recommend you take a vitamin supplement to ensure you're getting the recommended daily amounts of each vitamin. This is very common for the person who is trying to lose weight and is on a relatively low-calorie diet.

Minerals are inorganic elements found in nature; the term *minerals* is generally reserved for those elements that are solid. Humans consume minerals in both the plant and animal food products they eat as well as the water they drink. Minerals are important for two reasons: (1) They are used as the building blocks for body tissues such as bone, muscle, and teeth and (2) many minerals are enzymes that aid in the body's metabolic processes. There are essential and non-essential minerals that our bodies need for these different processes. The essential nutrients must be taken in by ingestion of food or dietary supplements, since the body doesn't naturally produce these nutrients. However, non-essential minerals are produced by the body naturally; thus they do not have to be added to our daily dietary intake. Inadequate mineral nutrition can be associated with various human diseases, so proper intake of the essential minerals (those not produced in the human body) is necessary for optimal health and physical performance [1].

Vitamin and Mineral Recommendations for Healthy Adults

Vitamin/Mineral	Dietary Reference Intakes (DRI)
B1/thiamin	1.2 mg
B2/riboflavin	1.3 mg
Niacin	16 mg
B6	1.7 mg
B12	2.4 mcg
Folic acid	400 mcg from food or 200 mcg synthetic
Biotin	30 mcg
Pantothenic acid	5 mg
C	90 mg
A	900 mcg/3000 IU
D	15 mcg/600 IU
E	15 mg
K	120 mcg
Calcium	1300 mg
Iron	18 mg
Phosphorus	1250 mg
Iodine	150 mcg
Magnesium	420 mg
Zinc	11 mg
Selenium	55 mcg
Copper	0.9 mg
Manganese	2.3 mg
Chromium	35 mcg
Molybdenum	45 mcg

Key: mg = milligrams; mcg = micrograms; IU = international units.

Source: From Center for Responsible Nutrition [2].

Special consideration should be paid to the bariatric (weight-loss) surgery patient when dealing with vitamin and mineral supplementation. The daily dietary recommended intake (DRI) for each remains the same as the non-surgical weight-loss person, but the surgical patient should take supplements for life, regardless of their dietary intake, because after surgery the patient's stomach is no longer able to absorb nutrients as well as it did before surgery. This malabsorption, which results from the surgical rearrangement of the intestinal tract, is especially prominent in gastric bypass patients. For maximum absorption of supplements, close attention should be paid to the most effective route for absorption and optimal dosage intervals. It is not uncommon for a bariatric patient to require a specific prescribed dose of a particular vitamin or mineral based on laboratory results.

WEIGHT-LOSS SURGERY DIETARY RECOMMENDATIONS

Individuals who have had weight-loss surgery must pay very special attention to their diet to ensure the success of the surgical procedure. Specific guidelines vary, depending on the surgeon. If you have had weight-loss surgery, always consult with your surgeon if you have any questions or concerns about your diet. Some general guidelines follow.

RULES OF THUMB

- Do not drink fluids with meals. If you do, you will not feel full or satisfied because this essentially washes the food through the pouch (small "new" stomach).
- Eat slowly and chew your food thoroughly; do not try to swallow chunks of food.
- Eat small portions; learn to recognize satiety (satisfaction) instead of fullness.
- Avoid sugary foods.
- Avoid caloric beverages (e.g., Coke, sweet tea, Gatorade, alcoholic drinks).
- Try to keep your meals protein rich; be sure to select lean proteins.
- Eat only when you are hungry. Just because it is lunch time doesn't mean you have to eat lunch. It is important to recognize the physical sensation of hunger before you eat. Sometimes we think we're hungry, but usually we're just bored. Recognize true hunger!

Understanding and Building on the Four Pillars of Fitness

- Keep a journal of your food intake for the first month or two following surgery and do so again whenever you're having trouble sticking with your dietary plan.
- Take a multivitamin daily. Make sure it contains vitamin B12, calcium, iron, and folic acid.

Recommended Macronutrient Percentage

Carbohydrate = 40% of total caloric intake	Fat = 30% of total caloric intake	Protein = 30% of total caloric intake
The majority consisting of complex carbs	The majority coming from mono- & polyunsaturated fats	The majority coming from lean meats & low-fat dairy products
1 gram of carb = 4 calories	1 gram of fat = 9 calories	1 gram of protein = 4 calories

SAMPLE WEIGHT-LOSS DIET ACCORDING TO RECOMMENDED MACRONUTRIENT PERCENTAGE

1,600 Calorie Diet Consisting of 40 Percent Carbohydrate, 30 Percent Protein, 30 Percent Fat

This sample diet was created and provided by a registered dietician, Nichole Ulibarri, MS, RD. In addition, Nichole personally reviewed and approved all dietary recommendations in this chapter. This sample diet is based on 1,600 calories daily. The number of servings is noted in parentheses behind each meal or snack option. Depending on your metabolism and daily activity, you may need to increase or decrease this caloric amount in order to lose weight. Keep in mind that a loss of 1-2 lb per week is considered healthy weight loss and that there are 3,500 calories in 1 lb of fat. Therefore, if you create a weekly caloric deficit of 3,500 calories, you should lose about 1 lb each week. Similarly, if you create a weekly deficit of 7,000 calories, you should lose about 2 lb each week.

BREAKFAST

Omelet: Make an omelet in a skillet with non-stick cooking spray, using 2 egg whites, 1 ounce of shredded 2-percent milk cheese, and 1 cup assorted chopped vegetables (e.g., tomatoes, mushrooms, onions, or broccoli). Add 2 slices of reduced calorie whole wheat toast topped with 1 tsp margarine. (2 ounces meat, 1 carbohydrate, 1 non-starchy vegetable, 1 fat)

SNACK

6 ounce light yogurt and 1/3 cup each of blueberries, raspberries, and strawberries (1 ounce meat, 2 carbohydrate)

LUNCH

Tuna boats: Mix together 1 can/pouch water-packed tuna, 1 Tbsp reduced-fat mayonnaise, ½ cup each of chopped cucumber and celery. Add salt, pepper, and vinegar as desired. Spoon mixture onto 2 tomato halves and serve with 1 slice of whole wheat pita bread. (3 ounces of meat, 2 carbohydrates, 2 non-starchy vegetables, 1 fat)

SNACK

3 cups air-popped popcorn (1 carbohydrate)

DINNER

Stir-fry: Cook 4 oz of skinless chicken pieces in skillet. Add 3 cups mixed vegetables (bock choy, broccoli, snap peas, bean sprouts, carrots, red peppers, onions, and water chestnuts). Cook with 1 tsp oil and 1 Tbsp soy-sauce until vegetables are tender. Add water if more steam is needed. Serve with 2/3 cup steamed brown rice. (3 ounces meat, 3 non-starchy vegetables, 2 carbohydrates)

SNACK

1 stick of string cheese and 5 reduced-fat whole wheat crackers (1 ounce meat, 1 carbohydrate)

REFERENCES

1. Williams, Melvin, H. *Nutrition for Health, Fitness & Sport*, 6th Ed. New York: McGraw-Hill, 2002. Pp 14, 139, 146-151, 275.
2. Center for Responsible Nutrition. Source for vitamin and mineral DRI's. Available at: www.cmusa.org; accessed November 28, 2008.

Chapter 5
Getting Started with Exercise

Now that you have embraced the idea of a lifestyle change to become physically active, have identified your fitness environment, understand and accept your physical limitations, understand the four pillars of fitness, and are motivated to get started, you just need to know how to begin to achieve your fitness goals. This is where people tend to get themselves in trouble.

Sometimes, we are so motivated to get started that we do way too much, far too fast. It's like making too many rash New Year's resolutions. Let's say it is January 1, and you have made the decision to get fit in the next year. Despite the fact that you haven't exercised for several months or possibly years, you decide that you need to really do it right this time. So you start exercising five days a week for 30-45 minutes a day. You start doing mostly cardiovascular exercise and throw in some strength training here and there. The strength training consists of your random choice of working out on three or four different weight machines, but you aren't exactly sure what muscle groups you are training. It is great that you started, but you could be far more successful with your exercise for weight loss if you had started more slowly and progressed less aggressively toward your goal.

It is important to understand that exercise is stress to your body. If you introduce too much stress too fast, your body will shut down. In other words, this approach will not result in appropriate weight loss, inches lost, change in body composition, increase in cardiovascular fitness, and muscular strength. This is quite a consequence! It underscores why it is so important to exercise the right way. When you experience too much stress, your body tends to become run down and fatigued; sometimes you get sick. The same can happen if you subject your body to too much exercise too quickly. The good news is that a moderate level of stress, especially moderate physical stress through exercise, promotes health and prevents physical deterioration. You just have to introduce the new stress of exercise in progressively appropriate amounts and not overdo the amount or intensity of exercise. There is such a thing as too much stress through exercise. Sometimes, too much stress on your body can be a result of being overly motivated to exercise. Let me tell you a story about an overly motivated client I had one time.

It was a Friday afternoon when Martha came into my office frantically looking for some help with her exercise. I am always excited to help clients, especially when they appear to be ready to help themselves. Martha sat down and feverishly explained how she was ready to get in shape and make a change. She further explained that she wanted to a hire a personal trainer. I told her we could definitely work together to help her make the change. She said, "I want a trainer who isn't going to be easy on me. I want somebody who is going to push me. I need a motivator, not someone who is going to let me slide every time I whine or complain about how it is too difficult."

"Not a problem," I told her, "but do understand that you do not want to do too much too soon, since it's been quite some time since you've been consistent with any exercise." She said, "Yeah, I hear you, but I have to get in shape now! I need somebody to push me, and I want to train at least four times a week, maybe more."

I told her I could help her, proceeded to sign her up for a training package, and scheduled her training sessions. She wanted to start the next day, so I set her up for an initial cardiovascular fitness assessment. The assessment she signed up for is called *VO2 indirect calorimetry*. This particular assessment evaluates overall cardiovascular fitness or heart health and reveals how efficient or inefficient the body is burning fat. The test generally lasts only about 15 minutes; however, it pushes a person to their maximal level of exertion. So I signed this particular client up for this service. She went on to explain how she was ready to get fit and she wanted to do an hour of personal training immediately following the test. I told her she could do the hour of personal training, but she should be cautious because if she did too much too soon, her body wouldn't react the right way. She said, "No, I need to do this, and I want to get started now."

Over the years, I've learned that, on occasion, you have to help your clients understand the positive and negative results of exercise and advise them how to proceed with an individualized program, based on their current level of fitness. Then, if they don't listen and insist on doing it their own way, they learn the hard way—through subsequent post-exercise pain and discomfort. So, I scheduled Martha for the next-day training session she insisted upon. As the saying goes in sales and customer service, "The client is always right," and a client seeking advice and guidance on an exercise program must initially be shown deference unless he/she could be injured or suffer real harm by stubbornly refusing that advice and guidance.

Martha came in the next day and performed her fitness assessment. This alone was quite challenging for her; she scored well below average on her cardiovascular fitness assessment. We reviewed all of the results and she proceeded to her training session. I had scheduled her with one of my staff who tends to "push" clients fairly hard. I spoke with the trainer the previous day to explain Martha's wishes. I also asked him to reiterate that she wouldn't be able to start off exercising too hard too soon and that if she did, she may end up with aches and pains that would be obstacles to progressing as she wished.

As she started her training session, she told the trainer once again her wish to be pushed really hard. After a bit of discussion, the trainer satisfied her request. About 30 minutes into a 1-hour session, she started to look pretty peeked. The trainer didn't ease up, since the client was still determined to get through the self-inflicted punishment. After a few more exercises, she finally relented and told my trainer she wasn't going to be able to complete the rest of the session. She said she was completely exhausted and couldn't continue. Having heard from her how much she wanted to be pushed to continue, the trainer was a bit surprised but certainly not shocked that she wanted to quit.

This is just one example of how important it is to understand how your fitness level dictates the appropriate intensity of your exercise workout. If the exercise intensity is inappropriately high for your level of fitness, it results in adverse effects on your body and on your motivation to press ahead. This particular client didn't even come back to finish her training sessions. Often, we are overzealous or maybe not quite ready to do what our brains want us to do. That is okay. Keep these initial desires intact, and set goals for yourself. If you start slowly and gradually progress, increasingly the intensity level of your exercise program appropriately as your fitness improves, you will meet and surpass your fitness and weight-loss goals.

In order to start exercising slowly and gradually progressing or increasing in intensity, remember to stay balanced on the four pillars of fitness discussed in the previous chapter: flexibility, cardio (aerobic) exercise, strength training, and a healthy diet. If you do, you will lose weight and meet your fitness goals at a faster rate. If you don't have the proper mix or balance of these four pillars of fitness (e.g., thinking back to the analogy of a table used in the previous chapter, one or more legs of the table is missing or shorter than the rest), you will tip over or fall short of your weight loss and fitness goals. You'll have a better chance at sticking to your exercise routine for the long run if you gradually progress, accomplishing each pillar of fitness in your exercise routine. Remember, this is a lifelong endeavor, not a single destination.

The best part of exercising is that you don't have to kill yourself to get fit. In fact, the most important factor in how much weight you lose is how consistent you are with your workouts, not the intensity of the workouts. In fact, an article in the Mayo Clinic Proceedings states, "Emphasis is moving away from intermittent sweat-drenched bouts of arduous exercise to more frequent walking, whether in the park, at work, or at home" [1].

RULES OF THUMB

General rules of thumb for starting an exercise program to lose weight and become more fit are:

- Start slowly and gradually progress.
- Make sure your exercise routine is well balanced on the four pillars of fitness discussed in the previous chapter (i.e., flexibility exercise, cardio exercise, strength training, and a healthy diet).
- If you haven't exercised for several months or even years, make sure you don't overdo it and start with cardiovascular exercise and then add some form of strength training three to four weeks after starting your exercise routine.
- Do not skip exercising for more then two consecutive days. In other words, don't take three straight days off from your exercise routine. You can actually lose nearly 50 percent of your aerobic capacity by taking a whole week off from aerobic exercise, so be consistent with your workouts!
- Perform initial assessments to understand your current fitness level and help you set up your initial exercise program. If you're in poor physical shape, start exercising very slow and at low levels of intensity and duration. If you're in

fairly good physical shape, you can start exercising more frequently and at a moderate level of intensity.
- Track your progress. Once you've set initial goals, you should track your progress as you proceed in your exercise program. A lot of things can be tracked, the important thing is to ensure you understand how you are doing and where you are at with your weight loss and overall fitness goals. Here are some key ways to track your progress:
  1. Take pictures of yourself each month so that you can see how much weight you've lost.
  2. Track your pounds and inches lost.
  3. Laboratory results are also important to track; this data may have to be obtained from your physician's office. Improvement in lab results are rewarding because you can see how your efforts are positively impacting your health as well as your weight loss.
  4. Many people keep a journal of their food intake to ensure they're staying on track with their diet. If you're having emotional struggles, it is very helpful to record your feelings in a journal. This may reveal the reason for the emotional struggle.
- Do not overtrain. If you are exercising for two or more hours on most days of the week, you're overtraining unless you are training for an event or competition. If you are currently exercising for two or more hours on most days and you aren't training for a competition, you need to consult your physician or fitness professional.

CARDIO EXERCISE

- Generally speaking, low-to-moderate intensities of exercise burn more fat; however, this is relative to your fitness level. The more fit you are, the better your body burns fat at higher intensities and longer durations. This is why you need to exercise in order to lose weight! This is also why you need to increase your intensity levels as you become more fit. You can't stay at low to moderate intensities forever, but this is definitely the right place to start.
- If your weight or other limitations prevent you from doing cardio exercise, you may need to start with some basic strength-training activities such as seated, chair exercises until you lose some weight. Losing weight will allow you to do cardio exercise.
- Track your heart rate when you do your cardio. If you know your different training zones, be sure to start in the fat-burning zone and then progress the

intensity level according to your weight loss and increased fitness level. To learn more about measuring your heart rate and determining your fat-burning zone, see Chapter 7.
- Gradually build up the duration (in time) and frequency (in days) of your cardio exercise. If you can build up to doing 1 hour of cardio exercise six days of the week, this will be very effective in promoting weight loss.
- After about three to four months, incorporate interval training into your routine. Interval training specific to cardio is basically training at different intensities for different periods of time. For example, to incorporate interval training into a 30-minute walk, walk at a steady state for 7 minutes and then increase your speed to a serious power walk for 3 minutes. Repeat this: Return to your normal walking speed for 7 minutes and power walk again for 3 minutes. Do this sequence for three cycles or for a total of 30 minutes. In tracking your heart rate, you should be able to walk for 7 minutes at a relatively low heart rate and then increase your speed for 3 minutes to get your heart rate up to 10-20 beats per minute (bpm)—that is, if your heart rate is 90 bpm during the slow 7-minute walk, speed up enough to increase your heart rate to 110 bpm for the next 3 minutes. Again, repeat 7- and 3-minute cycles for a total of 30 minutes of exercise. Refer to Chapter 7 or check with your fitness professional to determine your exact heart-rate training zones.
- Remember that cardio exercise is best for weight loss, especially loss of fat pounds, so don't skip your cardio sessions.

STRENGTH TRAINING

The main objective of strength training is to maintain your lean muscle mass through the weight-loss phase. In other words, you shouldn't be trying to increase the size of your muscles if your primary objective is weight loss. If you try to do this, weight loss will be a little slower at first; essentially, you'll be adding muscle underneath the fat. You'll want to delay building muscle mass (size) until after you've attained your weight-loss goal. Then you can incorporate muscle toning, building, and sculpting.

- Initially, you should perform two or three sets of 12-20 repetitions for your strength-training exercises. This method of training is most advantageous for weight loss, and it prevents muscle hypertrophy. Muscle hypertrophy occurs when you increase the size of your muscles, which will subsequently increase your weight. Muscle hypertrophy may result from lifting heavier weight through lower repetitions (e.g., 4-6 reps).

- Use light to moderately heavy weights. Keep the exercise sets between one and three, and the repetitions between 12 and 15. In other words, if you perform one set of 12-15 repetitions and feel that you could probably perform four or five more repetitions with the that particular weight, you should select a heavier weight for the second set. Essentially you want to be able to complete the full number of repetitions (12-15) with good form and struggle a bit with the last two repetitions. If it is still easy when you complete the full number of repetitions, you should select a heavier weight for that particular exercise. The reverse is true if you're unable to complete the full number of repetitions; select a lighter weight in this instance.
- Do not perform exercises that work the same muscle group in consecutive order. For example, you should not perform a dumbbell bicep curl immediately followed by a dumbbell hammer curl or perform a chest press followed by a pushup. This style of training may cause muscle hypertrophy, which is not the initial goal for a weight-loss client. Organize your strength-training routine in such a way that each exercise works a different muscle group: for example, a chest press followed by a seated row exercise.
- If you strength train, never train the same muscle groups on consecutive days. This can cause severe muscle soreness and muscle injury.
- You can do cardio exercise on consecutive days but always rest for a full day each week or at least do not perform a structured workout one day a week. It doesn't really matter which day you take off; pick a day that best fits your schedule.

FLEXIBILITY EXERCISES

- Always spend 5-10 minutes stretching after a workout.
- Hold your stretches for 10-30 seconds.
- Do not stretch to the point of pain; you should feel a slight yet comfortable pull on the muscles during the stretch.

DIETARY AND HYDRATION GUIDELINES

- Eat small portions and a variety of foods frequently throughout the day (at least four to six times per day).
- Low-carbohydrate and high-protein diets (i.e., lean protein) are most advantageous to your weight-loss goals.
- Include whole-grain foods and avoid foods that rapidly spike your blood glucose or fall in the high range on the glycemic index.
- Drink plenty of water: Eight to 10 glasses of water (approximately 8 ounces per glass) daily is recommended. However, many factors can influence the need to increase your intake of water. Being more active, fighting an illness, or living in a hot and humid environment, for example, may require that you drink more water each day.
- Set initial goals and make sure they are realistic and achievable. To be realistic and achievable, your goals must be set on the basis of your current condition. Losing 10 lb in three weeks may be an initial goal; losing a total of 5 inches in two months may be another goal; walking for five consecutive minutes may be yet another. The point is that it is important to set initial concrete goals that you can achieve and that help you understand what you're striving for. If the only goal you set is a general, ambitious one—for example, to lose 150 lb—you may become very frustrated along the way, since this will take quite a long time to accomplish safely, without risking injury and medical problems. Set smaller, achievable milestone goals so that you can periodically measure your progress and be motivated by your accomplishments along the way. This will help you continue to strive toward achieving your ultimate goal. One initial goal I've seen many physicians set for overweight patients is a loss of 10 percent of their current body weight. This is an initial goal that is realistic and achievable.

REFERENCE

1. Levine, James A. Exercise: a walk in the park? *Mayo Clinic Proceedings* 2007;82(7)(July):797.

Chapter 6
Understanding and Accepting Your Limitations: Exercising Without Injury

Limitations? What limitations? You're ready to lose weight and you're not going to let anything stop you. Wow! I love that attitude. You may be doing your best to prevent anything from standing in your way; however, it is important to recognize that many people have physical limitations and/or medical conditions that can affect their ability to perform certain exercises, and you may be one.

A limitation is just that—a limitation. It doesn't mean you can't work out. As long as you understand your limitations and know how to work around them, they won't get in the way of your goals, that is, weight loss and improved health. This is why it is important to ensure your exercise program is free from risks for injury, because an injury could set you back in your efforts to lose weight and lead to overall frustration and anger.

Over the years, I've had clients with the attitude that they are not going to let anything get in their way, but I've also had clients who were very nervous about starting an exercise program for fear of injuring themselves. Many with physical limitations or medical conditions especially fear that exercise might cause injury that would further restrict their current activity levels. This may be the main reason why they have been inactive for several years.

Individuals who fear exercise are actually exciting to work with as clients because once they start exercising, they invariably feel better and their ability to move and get around in life improves. The more sedentary you are, the less cooperative your joints. It's kind of like the old tool that sits in your garage for years on end without use: After several years, the tool becomes rusty and difficult to use. Your body works the same way; we've all heard the expression "Use it or lose it." This is so true regarding the human body. The key is to know what to do and what not to do in order to keep your body moving in the" right direction," free from injury.

This chapter discusses different exercise movements and issues for you to keep in mind, depending on the type of limitation or medical condition you may have. Awareness of some of the contraindicated movements specific to your condition will help you avoid injury. However, also keep in mind that if you are limited by some type of condition, you may need to strengthen the muscles around the affected joint by doing some rehabilitative exercises. Incorporate these rehabilitative exercises into your regular exercise program. These types of exercises should help you significantly because if you continue to avoid physical activity, you risk becoming more and more debilitated—that is, your body may become weaker and your limitations may increase.

RULES OF THUMB

- If you have joint pain, avoid the exercise that itself produces pain in a particular joint.
- If you experience discomfort or pain in a muscle due to a particular exercise or activity, it is generally safe to continue except, of course, if you injured the muscle itself.
- Unless a doctor has specifically directed you *not* to exercise due to a physical limitation or medical condition, you can rest assured that exercise can improve the limitation or condition, provided you know what exercises are appropriate.

Maybe you're not sure if you have a limitation. How do you know what your limitation is? First, you need to go through a little bit of health history to identify any medical conditions or previous injuries you have experienced in the past.

Are there certain activities that cause pain to your joints? If so, you more than likely have a joint limitation. Maybe you have a medical condition that could be affected by exercise, such as diabetes, asthma, a heart condition, cancer, fibromyalgia, muscular dystrophy, arthritis, multiple sclerosis, or osteoporosis. The good thing is that if you do have any of these conditions, exercise will help you feel better, provided you know what you are doing. If you don't know what you are doing, exercise could cause your condition or limitation to worsen. This is why it is important to understand exactly what types of exercise to avoid as well as which specific exercises will help your condition, foster weight loss, and promote overall fitness and health.

A number of exercise restrictions or limitations for specific conditions are subsequently discussed in this chapter. Identify what, if any, condition (i.e., physical limitation or medical condition limitation) you have and then go to that section to review the guidelines for exercise and other suggestions as to what you should and shouldn't do. (Sections are in alphabetical order.)

ARTHRITIS

Arthritis is inflammation of a joint or joints, usually accompanied by pain, swelling, and stiffness. If you have arthritis, you have good days and bad days (days when an affected joint is inflamed). If a joint is inflamed, avoid exercising the affected area, especially if you have rheumatoid arthritis. In addition, follow these exercise guidelines:

- Always begin slowly and progress gradually.
- Focus on the following exercise goals if you have arthritis:
  1. Improve your muscular strength to keep joints stable.
  2. Improve your joint flexibility.
  3. Enhance your cardiovascular/aerobic fitness.
  4. Protect the affected joint(s).
  5. Alleviate pain.
- If you have arthritis, stretching and increasing your overall flexibility is critical to keep your muscles long and flexible. If you never stretch your muscles, they tend to shorten in length. When your muscles become short or tight, they pull on your arthritic joints, causing more pain. Stretching helps alleviate muscle tightness; this, in turn, decreases pain and improves the functionality of the joint due to the increased range of motion.
- Keep your aerobic training at a relatively low intensity and low impact. As you become stronger, you'll need to gradually increase the intensity in order to increase your cardiovascular fitness.
- Be sure to include a variety of cardiovascular exercises such as walking, biking, or swimming. Swimming is ideal for people with severe arthritis due to the low impact a water environment offers; low-impact puts less stress on the joints.

- Strength training improves the strength of the muscles. This, in turn, lessens the stress on the joints because the strengthened muscles around the joints take over some of the weight bearing from the joints. Your exercise routine should consist of one to three sets of 10-12 repetitions, depending upon the severity of the arthritis. There are three general rules to follow:
  1. Keep your strength-training exercises low impact.
  2. If you're a beginner, use of weight machines is usually best when you initially start your exercise regimen.
  3. Perform exercises that do not put additional strain on the joint(s) affected by your arthritis.

BREAST CANCER

Prevention of lymphedema is very important for breast cancer patients and other cancer patients who have had lymph nodes removed. Lymphedema is a swelling produced by an accumulation of lymph fluid in the tissue. If you have or have had breast cancer and underwent a lumpectomy or mastectomy procedure, it is very important to know how to prevent and identify lymphedema. A lumpectomy is the removal of a tumor and some lymph nodes from a woman's (or man's) breast, which is generally followed by radiation. Mastectomy is surgical removal of an entire breast or both breasts. Lymph nodes are generally removed during this procedure.

If you've had a lumpectomy or mastectomy, follow these guidelines for preventing lymphedema:

- Avoid any skin irritations (e.g., insect bites, hang nails, cuts).
- Avoid extreme water temperatures, both hot and cold.
- Wear a compression sleeve on the affected arm/side to avoid pooling of fluid. This is also recommended if you are traveling in an aircraft.
- Do not overdo it when you start to exercise; start slowly and gradually progress.
- Track girth measurements of the arm on the affected side, especially before and after exercise. This is done by measuring the circumference of your arm in four places (wrist, half way between your wrist and elbow, elbow, half way between your elbow and shoulder) before and after exercise. If there is a change in the measurement of a portion of your arm that is greater than or equal to ½ inch after you exercise, see a physician.

CANCER (ALL)

If you have or have had cancer, the goals of exercise therapy vary, depending on your status as a cancer patient. Are you in initial treatment, in remission, or in treatment for recurrence. Although exercise is very beneficial for individuals battling cancer, you'll need to understand and evaluate your current condition and individualize your exercise accordingly. For example, if you recently underwent chemotherapy or radiation sessions, chances are that you won't feel up to doing much exercise. In this case, you may stick to stretching or very short, low-intensity cardio workouts. Although cancer therapy—namely, chemotherapy and radiation therapy—causes fatigue, regular exercise appears to reduce fatigue as well as improve mood and enhance body image.

The main exercise goals are:

- Improving your strength and endurance.
- Managing your weight.
- Regaining your ability to perform routine daily activities. All cancer survivors should strive to return to a healthy, active lifestyle and incorporate regular exercise into their lifestyle.

If you have or have had cancer, follow these exercise guidelines [1]:

- Perform cardio and strength-training sessions at a low to moderate intensity and be aware of any adverse symptoms you experience during or after your exercise sessions.
- Perform flexibility exercises daily. This is especially important if you are undergoing or have undergone radiation therapy, because the radiation can cause a loss of flexibility.
- Perform aerobic exercise three or four times per week for 15-40 minutes in duration.
- Incorporate strength training two or three times per week, keeping the sessions to about 30 minutes in duration.
- Do not over do it; start slow and gradually progress.

DIABETES

Diabetes is a disease characterized by excess glucose (sugar) in the blood. It is a metabolic autoimmune disease, meaning that the body's immune system is malfunctioning, causing improper metabolism of glucose circulating in the bloodstream. Glucose is the main component of the food we ingest and is basically the body's fuel, providing the body with energy and "propelling" it in the activities it performs.

There are two primary types of diabetes: type I, also referred to as *insulin-dependent diabetes*, and type II, also called *non-insulin-dependent diabetes*, *insulin-resistant diabetes*, or *adult-onset diabetes*. A detailed discussion of the underlying cause, and the resulting abnormality in glucose metabolism, involved in each of the two types is very complex and beyond the scope of this book, but a simplified explanation of the two types follows:

- *Type I diabetes:* Type I diabetics are insulin dependent, meaning they require the injection of insulin at regular intervals during any 24-hour period because the body (specifically the pancreas) does not produce any insulin, which is crucial for the metabolism of glucose. Essentially, the body's immune system has gone awry and destroyed the pancreas' insulin-producing cells. Type I is much less common than type II, affecting less than 10 percent of all people with diabetes [2], but its medical management is considerably more difficult and complex because of the wider swings in the blood glucose levels throughout the day. These wide swings (the highs and lows) in the level of glucose in the blood put type I diabetics at greater risk for life-threatening complications due to severe hypoglycemia (low blood glucose) and hyperglycemia (high blood glucose). In addition, the necessity of regular insulin injections throughout the day at variable doses (depending on the blood glucose level at the particular time a glucose-monitor reading is done) usually make management of type I diabetes and its symptoms more complex and challenging.
- *Type II diabetes:* Type II diabetes has a different underlying cause but produces essentially the same symptoms and medical complications as type I diabetes if the disease is untreated. In type II diabetes, although the pancreas produces insulin, the body has become resistant to the insulin secreted by the pancreas and therefore cannot *use* it for the metabolism of glucose. Type II diabetes is usually somewhat easier to manage effectively than type I.

For many (but not all) type II diabetics, oral medication is effective and insulin injections are not required.

Classic symptoms of diabetes include extreme thirst, unexplained fatigue, blurry vision, and rapid, unexplained weight loss or weight gain.

If you are diabetic, you'll need to work closely with your doctor to treat and monitor the disease and its symptoms. Your physician will use a combination of the following medical management options: oral medication, meal planning, insulin injections, weight loss, and physical activity. You should be very aware of your blood glucose levels at all times. Therefore, you must understand and perform daily periodic self-monitoring of your blood glucose levels using a glucometer. If you measure too-high or too-low blood glucose levels or experience the more severe symptoms of diabetes for more than a day, you should schedule an appointment with your doctor as soon as possible.

Because both types of diabetes are metabolic disorders, effective disease and symptom management requires not only oral medication or insulin (or a combination of each is some cases), but also (1) strict dietary measures, (2) careful meal planning, involving eating on a regular schedule and ingestion of the right foods, and (3) regular exercise. These three lifestyle measures (modifications), in addition to oral medication or insulin injections, are crucial in making the body's metabolism of glucose work efficiently, maintaining a healthy weight, preventing disease symptoms, and avoiding potentially serious complications of the disease (i.e., retinopathy, neuropathy, dehydration, poor circulation, cardiovascular disease). All three modifications work together synergistically, "as a team," and are essential for diabetics to make in their lifestyle. You can think of these three lifestyle measures (modifications) like the legs of a tripod, all necessary to stabilize the disease.

DIETARY RESTRICTIONS

The main dietary restrictions for diabetics, whether they are type I or type II, are basically the same as the dietary guidelines detailed in Chapter 4 and they are even more important for effective weight loss and overall health. In fact, they are essential for control of the disease and its symptoms. Some foods contain more glucose than others and, if not avoided or eaten in small quantities, can cause serious diabetes-related symptoms and medical complications.

MEAL PLANNING AND SCHEDULING

If you are a diabetic, you need to eat meals on a regular schedule and eat the right foods in the proper proportions (restricting those with high amounts of glucose). You may also need to eat a protein snack like a beef jerky stick or a cup of low-fat cottage cheese in between meals to stabilize your blood glucose level.

EXERCISE

Like a proper diet and meal planning, regular exercise is critical for both type I and type II diabetics. Exercise basically acts like insulin by promoting the efficient metabolism of glucose, the body's fuel. Since exercise is a critical component of disease management for both type I and type II diabetics, the following exercise guidelines are very important:

GENERAL GUIDELINES

- Always have a rapidly absorbed carbohydrate (preferably over-the-counter glucoses tablets) with you, wherever you exercise, in case you become hypoglycemic (lower than normal blood glucose level—that is, less than 80 mg/dL).
- When you first begin an exercise program, do not overdo the duration or the intensity of the exercise.
- Because diabetics are prone to slow-healing wounds and skin infections, especially on the lower extremities, pay close attention to the condition of your feet. Proper foot care is important to prevent blisters, cuts and open sores, and ulcers. Therefore, it is very important to:
  1. Perform daily foot inspections. Look for any red spots, blisters, or open sores. Also, examine your feet for any imbedded foreign objects or insect bites.
  2. Perform proper foot hygiene. Wash your feet daily. Keep them clean and use lotion to prevent dry skin or cracking of the heels.
  3. Wear shoes and socks that are comfortable and not too tight. Some people use lotion or Vaseline on their feet to prevent rubbing (friction) on their feet, which may cause blisters, open sores, or ulcers. In diabetics, skin lesions, especially if they occur on a foot or leg, are often slow and difficult to heal due to decreased circulation in the extremities as a result of the disease.
  4. Neuropathy (nerve pain and numbness) in the upper and lower extremities is a possible complication of diabetes. If you suffer from neuropathy in

- the lower extremities, depending on its severity neuropathy, you may have stepped on a sharp object, such as a nail, and not have even realized it. If you are a diabetic with neuropathy, you must practice special vigilance in making sure your feet are free from injury.
- Over time, regular exercise combined with a change in eating habits may reduce the severity of type II diabetes and its adverse physical effects. As type II diabetics continue to exercise and lose weight, they may need to lower their medication dosage but should never do so without consulting their physician. (In some cases, type II diabetics who make the three necessary lifestyle changes may arrest the disease and no longer require medication.) Type I diabetics, who require insulin injections, may need to adjust the amount of insulin used at each injection as they progress in their exercise program and dietary changes.

PRE-EXERCISE GUIDELINES

- Perform glucose self-monitoring of your blood glucose level, using your glucometer, before each exercise session. Ideal pre-exercise blood glucose levels are between 100 and 180 mg/dL.
- If the glucometer reading of your blood glucose level is greater than 200 mg/dL and you have ketones in your urine *or* your blood glucose level is greater than 300 mg/dL (regardless of ketone status), postpone exercise and contact your physician. Pharmacies carry several over-the-counter (non-prescription) products that you can use to test your urine for ketones. Basically you dip a test strip into the urine and then compare the results to a chart that is provided in the test kit.
- If your blood glucose level is less than 100 mg/dL, you may need to eat a low-glucose snack (for example, 4 ounces of orange juice, an apple, half a banana, or half of a sandwich made of whole wheat bread with unsweetened fruit spread) before you begin your exercise workout, since hypoglycemia may occur during or shortly after exercise because of the insulin-like glucose-reducing effects of exercise.
- Always warm up (perform light cardio or callisthenic movements) for about 10 minutes before you begin your workout.
- Carry medical information or identification with you such as a medical ID wrist band, necklace, or dog tags.

DURING EXERCISE

- At each exercise session, always start slowly and gradually increase the intensity of the session.
- If you have retinopathy (an eye condition that may occur as a complication of diabetes), do not lift anything over your head.
- Hydrate (drink water) every 15 minutes during exercise. Adequate hydration is critical for diabetics.
- During each exercise session, keep a rapidly absorbed carbohydrate (preferably over-the-counter glucose tablets) readily available in the event you develop symptoms of hypoglycemia, namely, dizziness, weakness, and/or blurred vision.
- If exercise is of long duration (greater than 60 minutes), you should test your blood glucose level during the exercise, and an additional 15-30 grams of carbohydrate may need to be eaten every hour [3].

POST-EXERCISE GUIDELINES

- After each exercise session, cool down slowly by doing 5-10 minutes of stationary stretching exercises.
- If you are a beginner in doing regular exercise, you may feel a bit fatigued two to three hours after each workout session. However, understand that post-exercise fatigue will not be a long-term effect as you progress in your program of exercise; in the beginning your body is simply adapting to the new stress of exercise. In fact, once your body adapts, you'll have more energy than ever before.

FIBROMYALGIA

This condition is characterized by chronic fatigue and muscle soreness. It is often coupled with depression and is more prevalent in women than men. Due to the ongoing fatigue and muscle soreness, exercise can seem challenging for someone with fibromyalgia. The good news is that exercise can actually help combat fatigue and decrease overall pain from the condition itself. One's stamina and overall well-being also improves with regular exercise. If you have fibromyalgia, follow these exercise guidelines:

- Exercise at low- to moderate-intensity levels.
- Focus on restoring and maintaining your functional ability to perform daily activities.

- Stick to low-impact exercises, especially in the beginning.
- Start slowly and gradually increase the frequency of your exercise regimen until you are exercising, on average, 30-60 minutes per day, but always allow for one day of rest.
- Strength training should consist of one to three sets, with 8-15 repetitions per set, two times a week.
- Avoid or limit eccentric motion—that is, motions in which you are resisting gravity. For example, if you are performing a bicep curl, the eccentric motion is the downward motion. If you are using some eccentric motion, be sure to shorten the time in that motion. If you have fibromyalgia, allow only 1-2 seconds performing the eccentric motion and 3 seconds in the concentric motion (the motion of contracting the muscles). Even though the eccentric motion is relatively fast, make sure the motion is controlled.
- If muscular pain increases, stop immediately.

HEART DISEASE

If you are a cardiac patient, seek exercise clearance from your cardiologist or primary care physician prior to starting any physical fitness program. Exercise training is relatively safe for the majority of cardiac patients who are appropriately assessed and cleared for undertaking an exercise program. However, it is best that your physician gives you clearance and outlines any specific limitations he/she requests that you follow. After you've received clearance from your cardiologist, adhere to the following exercise guidelines:

- Focus on cardiovascular fitness.
- Keep your heart rate less than 110 beats per minute (bpm) unless otherwise directed by your physician.
- With the guidance of your physician and/or fitness professional, set a safe upper-level training limit for your exercise program.
- Be aware of your overall rate of perceived exertion and intensity levels. In most instances, you should keep your rate of perceived exertion (RPE) less than 7. In other words, you should be able to carry on a conversation while exercising; your ability to talk may cause some effort or extra exertion in breathing, but you should still be able to talk. For more information regarding the intensity of your exercise, see the RPE scale in Appendix B.

- Use the following guidelines before starting a strength training program [4]:
  1. Do not start strength training for at least five weeks after the date of myocardial infarction or cardiac surgery. Cardiac patients should be involved in a cardiopulmonary rehabilitative program during these five weeks.
  2. Most people can carry up to 30 lb at three weeks after acute myocardial infarction; thus, strength training could be incorporated sooner but must be cleared by your physician.
  3. Make sure you are breathing properly and avoid any Valsalva maneuvers (i.e., holding your breath and blowing out).
- If you have hypertrophic cardiomyopathy (if you're not sure, ask your doctor), follow these guidelines:
  1. Obtain additional exercise clearance from your cardiologist or primary care physician.
  2. Limit physical activity to aerobic exercise and noncompetitive sports (if you plan to be engaged in sports).
  3. Avoid anaerobic exercise (e.g., strength training or high-intensity sprints) unless you have clearance from your cardiologist.

HIP OR KNEE REPLACEMENT

If you have had hip or knee replacement, chances are that you underwent the surgery to decrease pain and increase your mobility as well as improve the overall quality of your life. In order to maximize the benefits of hip or knee replacement surgery, it is imperative that you remain active. The key to remaining active is knowing what to do in order to prolong the life of your artificial joint. Here are some key exercise considerations:

- Check with your surgeon and/or physical therapist before beginning a regular exercise program.
- Start slowly and gradually increase the duration and frequency of your exercise regimen.
- Reduce the wear on your new joint to improve the long-term results of your total joint replacement. Consider the following information on joint wear and longevity of joint replacements:
  1. Technology has improved the longevity of joint replacements; however, very active people risk the possibility of requiring another surgery in 15-20 years.

2. Choosing aerobic activities with low joint load/impact, such as swimming, cycling, or possibly elliptical training, is recommended because these low-impact activities put less stress on the new joint.
- Focus on improving the strength of the muscles around the knee or hip joint, thus lessening the stress on the joint itself.

HIP REPLACEMENT

If you have had hip replacement, *avoid* the following exercises and/or movements:

- Crossing the midline of your body (i.e., do not cross your legs).
- Bending more than 90 degrees at the hip joint. This could cause dislocation of the newly replaced joint.
- High-impact activities such as jumping, running, or competitive sports.
- Activities that cause pain. Don't overdo it; any discomfort should be within reason.

Focus on increasing the range of motion and overall strength of the muscles surrounding the replaced knee or hip joint.

KNEE REPLACEMENT

If you have had knee replacement, *avoid* the following exercises and/or movements:

- Twisting your knee.
- High-impact activities such as jumping, running, or competitive sports.
- Activities that cause pain. Do not overdo it; you may feel a slight discomfort, but this discomfort should be reasonable.

HYPERTENSION (HIGH BLOOD PRESSURE)

You can find directions on how to assess your blood pressure in Chapter 8. The following section outlines blood pressure ranges relative to what exercise guidelines to consider if you have hypertension.

The following table shows the blood pressure categories and their corresponding systolic and diastolic blood pressure measurements (levels). The systolic measurement is the top number/value in your blood pressure reading, and the diastolic measurement is the bottom number/value.

Blood Pressure Categories

Blood Pressure Categories	Systolic Blood Pressure (mm Hg)	Diastolic Blood Pressure (mm Hg)
Optimal	Less than 120	Less than 80
Pre-hypertension	120-139	80-89
Hypertension	Greater than or equal to 140	Greater than or equal to 90

If your blood pressure reading falls in the range for the hypertension category but you don't have any cardiovascular disease, you are encouraged to participate in an exercise program. However, make sure your blood pressure is evaluated, treated, and monitored regularly by your physician. If you do have cardiovascular disease, it is very important that your physician clears you to exercise prior to starting any fitness program.

Exercise guidelines for people with hypertension are:

- Focus on cardiovascular activities that are low to moderate in intensity.
- Avoid Valsalva maneuvers (holding your breath and blowing out) during strength training.
- Because weight reduction and healthy eating habits are extremely important in helping reduce blood pressure, make losing weight the main goal of your exercise program.
- Set up your program to exercise 30-60 minutes a day on most days of the week; remember to always start slowly and gradually progress.
- Strength training should complement your aerobic training. Use light to moderately heavy weights. Keep the exercise sets between one and three, and the repetitions between 10 and 15.
- Do not exercise if your resting systolic (top value) blood pressure is greater than 200 mm Hg or your diastolic (bottom value) blood pressure is greater than 110 mm Hg. Again, refer to Chapter 8 to learn how to perform blood pressure measurement.

LUMBAR/CERVICAL BACK PROBLEMS

There are several different types, causes, and symptoms of back pain. Back pain can range from mild, dull, annoying pain to severe, excruciating, debilitating pain. Back pain appears to occur more frequently in the lumbar (lower) region of the back. If you are overweight or obese, the chance of experiencing back pain is essentially as sure as death and taxes, as the expression goes, because the excess weight you carry around automatically puts excessive strain on your low back. Eighty (80) percent of all people will experience back pain at some point in their lives. Back pain is the most common cause of inactivity for people under the age of 45, and costs associated with back pain are estimated to range from $50 billion to $100 billion annually [5]. This being said, we must find a way to combat back problems and rehabilitate those that suffer from back pain. If you suffer from back pain, follow these exercise guidelines:

- Make your primary fitness goals weight loss, pain reduction, improving posture and gait, increasing strength, and increasing flexibility and overall range of motion in the joints.
- Improve your core strength (i.e., strengthening the abdominal and back muscles). This is critical to managing low back pain because protecting the spine through increased strength of your core muscles ultimately reduces the strain on your spine.
- If you suffer from low back pain (lumbar and sacral), focus on improving the flexibility of the hip flexors, hamstrings, glutes, and core. If these muscles are tight, there is an increased risk for spasm of the back muscles due to increased tension on the lower back.
- If you suffer from upper back pain (cervical and thoracic), focus on improving the flexibility in the shoulders, neck, and upper back.
- Vary the intensity of the back and abdominal exercises based upon the level of pain. During acute pain, limit back and hip muscle exercises for two weeks and then gradually introduce low-intensity exercises.
- Avoid high-impact activities—that is, anything that will cause excess jarring of the spine such as competitive sports, jumping, or running.

LUMBAR OR CERVICAL DISC DISEASE (SPONDYLOSIS, DISC HERNIATION, BULGING DISC, OR SPINAL STENOSIS)

Lumbar or cervical disc disease, both more commonly referred to as *degenerative disc disease (DDD)*, is a natural part of our aging process. (*Lumbar* refers to the spine at the level of the back, and *cervical* refers to the spine at the level of the neck.) As we age, our intervertebral discs become less flexible and lose some of their ability to absorb shock, the ligaments around the discs may become stiff and brittle and the muscles surrounding the spine may weaken. In addition, the intervertebral discs may become compressed and the space around the nerve bundles may shrink. Bone spurs may also develop as a result of the disc compression. All these changes contribute to the onset of DDD and/or arthritis in the back, which ultimately causes back pain, leg pain, and weakness of the back.

If you suffer from DDD, follow these guidelines:

- Limit any movements that may cause further compression of the vertebrae—that is, limit flexion (bending) of the spine; loading (bearing of heavy weights) of the spine, depending on severity of your condition; and torsion (twisting) of the spine.
- If you have cervical disc disease, especially if you suffer cervical neck pain, limit any overhead lifting, as this causes compression of the spine and often forces the head or chin forward, creating more stress and strain on the neck/cervical spine.
- If pain is unrelenting or becomes severe, see your primary care provider.

MULTIPLE SCLEROSIS

The cause and disease progression of multiple sclerosis (MS) is beyond the scope of this book. If you have MS, I'm sure you know what it is, its symptoms, and how it can affect your daily life. However, you need to understand how it affects your exercise routine and your ability to be physically active.

Because MS directly affects the central nervous system, there are several symptoms that can limit your exercise. These symptoms include:

- Visual problems.
- Severe fatigue.
- Tendency to become overheated.

- Muscle weakness.
- Impaired mobility.
- Poor balance.
- Difficulty with coordination.

Because of these symptoms, especially the last four, it is important to incorporate strength training into your exercise program in an effort to minimize the risk of falling. Exercise can ease some of the symptoms of MS. Before you begin an exercise program, talk with your physician and follow any specific exercise guidelines or limitations he/she advises. In addition to your physician's recommendations, apply the following exercise guidelines to improve your fitness:

- Start slowly and gradually progress in your exercise regimen and, in each exercise session, be sure not to overdo it.
- Always warm up for 10 minutes before your workout and cool down for 5-10 minutes after an exercise session.
- Be sure to exercise in a safe environment, free of any tripping hazards.
- Do not become overheated; stay well hydrated and avoid outside activities during warm and hot weather.
- Keep a stabilizing object (e.g., chair, cane, wall) nearby if balance is an issue.

MUSCULAR DYSTROPHY

Muscular dystrophy is a hereditary disorder of the skeletal muscle system. It often leads to a progressive loss of strength and functional capacity. There are over 100 different types of muscular dystrophy. Some types of muscular dystrophy affect the heart, resulting in cardiomyopathy or arrhythmia (disturbance of the heart's rhythm).

Common symptoms of the disease, which may affect one's exercise regimen, are:

- Progressive muscular wasting or weakness.
- Poor balance.
- Frequent falling.
- Difficulty walking, including a waddling gait, or an inability to walk in some cases.
- Calf pain.
- Limited range of motion.

- Muscle contractures.
- Scoliosis (curvature of the spine).
- Drooping eyelids.

If you have muscular dystrophy, follow the guidelines listed below to help improve your fitness [3]:

- At each exercise session, stay well hydrated, do not overdo it, and always warm up for 10 minutes and cool down for 5-10 minutes.
- Start slowly and progress gradually, working up to 20-30 minutes of cardiovascular training for five to six days a week.
- Flexibility should be a primary focus of your exercise, as it helps to prevent contractures and loss of joint movement.
- For strength training, start by using a low weight and performing 10 repetitions. You need to use a weight that is about 25-30 percent of the total weight you could use to perform one repetition of the exercise; this is considered to be 25-30 percent of your 1-rep maximum.
- Over a period of weeks or months, gradually increase the weight you use for strength training.
- Be sure your exercise environment is safe—particularly that it is free from any tripping hazards.
- If you have a problem with balance, keep a stabilizing object (e.g., chair, cane, wall) close by so that you can grab it if necessary, or perform most of your exercise from a seated position.

OBESITY IN ADULTS

According to data collected in the National Health and Nutrition Examination Survey 2001-2004, nearly one in three U.S. residents are obese. In addition, there is evidence that low cardiovascular fitness increases the risk for death at a rate similar to the mortality rates associated with smoking, hypertension, and diabetes [6]. *Obesity* has been defined by many measurement systems, but the body mass index (BMI) scale is one tool generally used by physicians to diagnose a patient in a clinical setting. BMI is a value based on the ratio of your height and weight. It helps determine if an individual is obese, overweight, underweight, or of normal weight. Your BMI can be calculated by using a simple equation or a BMI chart. Specific guidelines on BMI calculation are given in Chapter 8. The following are standard BMI values for determining one's weight status:

- Normal weight: 18-24.9 BMI
- Overweight: 25-29.9 BMI
- Obesity class I: 30-34.9 BMI
- Obesity class II: 35-39.9 BMI
- Morbid obesity: 40 BMI or greater

Excess body weight generally restricts your ability to be physically active in one or more ways. The stress on your joints is one of the ways. Every day, your joints are withstanding a great amount of stress due to the excess weight they have to support. Therefore, weight loss is critical in order to reduce this stress. If your BMI is 30 or greater (i.e., if you are obese) and/or you haven't been physically active for quite some time, follow these physical activity recommendations:

- Increase your daily activity. For example, do the following to increase the amount of movement you perform during your daily or weekly routine: Wash your car, clean the house, park further away, try using the stairs instead of the elevator, walk to the mail box, stand instead of sitting, walk to your co-workers office instead of using e-mail all of the time.
- Start slowly and gradually increase your aerobic activity until you are exercising for 60 minutes a day, six days a week.
- If your BMI is greater than 35, protection of your joints is one of your most important concerns. Make every effort to avoid exercises that would create greater stress on your joints. Avoid activities such as jogging, jumping, and competitive contact sports.
- Do aerobic exercise that is low to moderate in intensity. This is best for weight loss.
- Emphasize duration over intensity in your aerobic exercise.
- Determine the severity of your obesity and select the method of exercise accordingly. For example, if you are 100 lb or more overweight, jogging or fast-paced walking is not recommended because it will create too much stress on your joints due to your excess weight. Similarly, if you're unable to walk

much (or not at all) because of your excess weight, perform all exercises from a seated position.
- Choose low-impact methods of exercise such as exercising in a pool, on a recumbent bike, or on an upper extremity bike.
- Strength training should consist of two or three sets of 12-15 repetitions—that is, do more reps per set and a relatively low number of sets and use light to moderately heavy weights. Your goal is not to bulk up your muscle mass, because this will cause weight gain rather than weight loss. You simply want to *maintain* muscle mass through the weight-loss phase; therefore, performing a higher number of repetitions is more advantageous to meeting your primary goal (weight loss). In addition, follow these strength-training guidelines:
  1. Lower body strength-training exercises may need to be geared more toward training on weight machines than using free weights. The reason for this is because your excess weight will cause some limitation in maintaining a normal center of gravity. If your center of gravity is off or shifted, it makes it much more difficult to perform lower body free-weight or functional exercises such as squats or lunges than to exercise on weight machines, which are stationary and thus provide stability. In addition, exercising on weight machines helps reduce stress on the knees.
  2. If you have major joint limitations in your lower extremities, try to perform most, if not all, of your strength exercises from a seated position.
  3. Before progressing to exercising with free weights, you'll need to lose some excess body weight and increase your strength and overall fitness.
- Obesity puts you at greater risk for injury because of the increased load on your joints and any additional conditions you may have as a result of your obesity. Therefore, it is important to remember (1) to always start slowly and then gradually increase your exercise and (2) to change up your exercise routine (i.e., flexibility, cardio, and/or strength) every four to six weeks.

OBESITY IN CHILDREN

Obesity is on the rise not only among adults but also among children. Some experts believe that if the rise in the obesity trend continues, the increase in life expectancy that has occurred around the world over the past century may come to a screeching halt. In fact, some speculate that kids may not outlive their parents. In an effort to reverse this trend in childhood obesity, it is important for kids to be physically active and start practicing healthy habits when they are young. If they don't, they may "become" one of the following alarming statistics:

- Over a 15-year period, childhood obesity increased over 50 percent [7], and lack of exercise accounts for over 50 percent of the cases of childhood obesity [8].
- Children who are not physically fit tend to have increased blood pressure and cholesterol, be more prone to type II diabetes, and acquire other chronic diseases [8].

Should children perform the same exercises as adults? What physical activities are healthy for children? These are all good questions. General exercise guidelines for children follow:

- Children, especially young children, should be involved in fun or game-like activities. Formal exercise is okay for adolescents, but younger children need more entertainment:
    1. Tag, jump rope, hide-and-seek, relays, sports, obstacle courses, etc., are all excellent exercise options for children.
    2. Watching television while doing different physical activities, group exercise, or different games may be helpful tactics to encourage young children to enjoy physical activity.
- Strength training can be very valuable for increased performance in sports, preventing injuries, and increasing the density of a child's bones. However, keep the following considerations in mind before starting a child in a strength training program:
    1. Generally speaking, if a child is old enough to be involved and participate in organized sports, he or she is old enough to participate in strength training and disciplined enough to follow directions and execute the proper lifting form involved to strength training. In addition, such a child is usually able to control the movements of his/her body more easily.
    2. A child should keep the lifting weight relatively light (i.e., approximately 65 percent of a child's one-rep maximum; this would equal about 65 percent of the total weight a child could lift one time for a particular exercise).
- A child should try to do at least 20-40 minutes of exercise each day. For weight loss, the child must gradually increase the duration of each exercise

session, working up to 60 minutes of physical activity on most days of the week. To achieve this goal, intermittent rounds of physical activity may be more realistic for some children.
- Parents should be involved in the following ways:
  1. They should be good role models; children tend to follow in their parents' footsteps.
  2. They should support and encourage their kids to practice healthy habits, including regular exercise and good eating habits.
  3. They should actively teach their children healthy eating habits. They should*n't prohibit* their kids from eating unhealthy foods, but simply allow these foods only in moderation.
  4. They should limit or reduce the amount of time their children are allowed to watch television, play on the computer, and play video games.
  5. If possible, they should encourage physical activity by making it a "family affair."

OSTEOPOROSIS/OSTEOPENIA

Many people develop osteoporosis or osteopenia as they grow older. Both conditions result from deterioration of the bone, causing it to become weak, fragile, and at risk of breaking. Osteoporosis can affect any bone, but the spine and the hips are of special concern because a fracture in either one of these areas can greatly affect one's ability to walk and to be active and thus may cause significant disability. A person is said to have osteopenia ("pre-osteoporosis") if the individual's bone density, or bone mass, is not low enough to be classified as osteoporosis but is low enough to be classified as being associated with greater risk of developing osteoporosis.

Regular exercise is one of the best ways to strengthen your bones and prevent osteoporosis and osteopenia. If you already have osteoporosis or osteopenia, exercise can help maintain the amount of bone-mineral mass (bone thickness) you have and can help arrest, or sometimes even reverse, the adverse effects of the disease. Exercising will help you attain the following important goals:

- Maintain joint stability.
- Improve coordination and balance.
- Reduce or prevent joint pain.
- Increase muscle strength.

- Prevent further loss of bone density (mass).
- Attain cardiovascular fitness.
- Maintain or improve posture and restore or maintain your general confidence.

If you have osteoporosis or osteopenia, follow these exercise guidelines:

- Begin slowly and gradually progress in your exercise regimen.
- *Absolutely avoid* (1) all high-impact activities, particularly competitive sports, and (2) all exercises that may load or bend the spine (e.g., a Smith machine squat, back extensions, lifting overhead). These types of exercise could cause fractures of the spine because they are loading the spine—that is, they put excess weight on the spine.
- To help keep your bones strong, try to do as much routine, daily weight-bearing exercises as possible (e.g., walking, stair climbing, vacuum cleaning). Performing these kinds of activities regularly helps stop further loss of bone density and weakening of the bones.
- Perform strength training, which generally should consist of two or three sets of 8-10 repetitions in each set. Use of weight machines rather than free weights is best for beginners. As you increase your strength, you may progress to use of free weights; however, consult a fitness professional to ensure you're executing free-weight exercises using proper form. This will help avoid injury.
- Do some low-impact cardio exercises, such as walking, bicycling, or swimming.
- Incorporate flexibility exercise such as stretching, yoga, or Tai Chi. Stretching helps to keep your joints flexible and encourages free range of motion; this will ultimately help prevent injury.
- Ensure the exercise surface is safe and free from any risk for falling.

PREGNANCY

If you are pregnant, understand that being pregnant doesn't preclude you from exercising, but you must minimize your risk of injury. In particular, you must avoid all contact sports. Methods of exercise you can do include walking, bicycling, swimming, low-impact aerobics, and strength training. Choose from among these activities. Exercise can make your pregnancy much more enjoyable and increase your comfort during this time. It may also make labor easier and less painful.

Exercising while pregnant produces many, if not all, of the following health benefits:

- Increased energy.
- Improved sense of well-being.
- Improved muscle tone.
- Increased strength.
- Greater endurance.
- Better posture.
- Appropriate weight gain.
- Faster recovery and shorter labor.
- Reduced back pain.
- Prevention of gestational diabetes.
- Easier adjustment to the demands of parenthood.

If you're pregnant, obtain clearance to exercise from your physician or health care provider. If you've received this clearance, follow these exercise recommendations:

- Exercise sessions should consist of 20-45 minutes. Try to perform these sessions three times a week.
- Keep the intensity of your exercise at a moderate level. Using the rate of perceived exertion (RPE) scale in Appendix B, try to restrict your exertion to approximately 3 or 4. At this level, you should be able to talk to someone nearby but conversation should require some effort. Another way to determine an appropriate, moderate level of exertion is to work out at about 50 percent of your maximum capacity. At 50 percent, the "talk test" should apply.
- Generally, your strength training should consist of two or three sets of 8-10 repetitions per set, and you should use light to moderate weights. Try to lift weights two times per week; three times per week is okay for more experienced exercisers.
- Avoid ballistic or high-impact movements, since your joints are more lax, or loose, due to the hormonal changes that occur during pregnancy.
- Avoid lunges and squats, since your center of gravity has shifted, making it more difficult to perform these movements and thus putting more stress on

your body. A lunge may also put your knee joint in a precarious position, since the hormonal changes cause the joint itself to be more unstable.
- During your second and third trimester, do not perform any exercises lying on your back and avoid long periods of standing in one position.
- During the third trimester, decrease the intensity and duration of your exercise. For strength training, it is important to use lighter weights, but you can perform an increased number of repetitions (10-15 reps).
- For the duration of your pregnancy, try to perform special exercises, such as Kegel and/or Hiss/Compress exercises, on a daily basis. These exercises help strengthen the pelvic floor, which in turn will help reduce the intensity and pain of contractions and make labor easier.
    1. Kegel exercises consist of contracting and relaxing the muscles that form part of the pelvic floor. Performing these exercises during pregnancy make delivery easier and can help prevent incontinence after giving birth. These exercises can also enhance women's sexual enjoyment.
    2. To perform Hiss/Compress exercises, sit on the floor with your legs gently crossed in front, centering your weight. Relax the abdomen and inhale; then exhale, compressing the abdomen and pulling the belly button toward the back of the spine. Slightly roll back and continue to compress the abdomen. Relax and repeat. This form of exercise is designed to help with discomfort during pregnancy and prepare you for labor.
- Stop exercising immediately if any of the following occur (these warning signs were established by the American College of Obstetricians and Gynecologists):

    1. Pain
    2. Vaginal bleeding
    3. Dizziness or feeling faint
    4. Rapid heartbeat
    5. Difficulty walking
    6. Uterine contractions
    7. Chest pain
    8. Fluid leaking from the vagina
    9. Insufficient weight gain
    10. Sudden swelling of ankles, hands, or face

SHOULDER INJURY

The shoulder is the most movable joint in the body; therefore, it is highly susceptible to injury. Common shoulder injuries include sprains, strains, bursitis, subluxation, dislocation, rotator cuff tears, frozen shoulder, tendonitis, fractures, and arthritis. Many people experience shoulder problems due to overuse or aging. If you think you have a shoulder injury, be sure to consult with your doctor prior to exercising. In addition, if shoulder pain persists for more than two weeks, consult your physician for further evaluation.

If you suffer a shoulder injury or are still trying to rehabilitate your shoulder after an injury, observe the following guidelines:

- Avoid any overhead lifting. This type of activity could cause more injury.
- Never lift or move your shoulder outside its normal range of motion: Raising your arm to the side or laterally above your shoulder is not a movement within the normal range of motion. This could cause nerve impingement or other damage to the shoulder joint. Such an adverse effect may not occur initially, but repetitive movements outside the normal range of motion can cause damage over time.
- Try doing different rehabilitative exercises to strengthen the shoulder capsule. Consult a fitness professional, athletic trainer, occupational therapist, or physical therapist for specific rehabilitative shoulder exercises.

WEIGHT-LOSS (BARIATRIC) SURGERY: GASTRIC BYPASS, OR ROUX-EN-Y (RNY), LAP-BAND, GASTRIC SLEEVE, OR DUODENAL SWITCH

To be covered for bariatric surgery, most insurance companies require an individual to have a BMI greater than 40 *or* greater than 35 as well as two or more co-morbidities (medical disorders associated with obesity).

Believe it or not, a weight-loss surgery patient does not have to observe very many exercise restrictions after the surgery because the surgical procedure allows the individual to be more physically active due to the ensuing, fairly rapid weight loss. The best thing you can do to prepare yourself both before and after surgery is to increase your fitness level. Recently, a study was performed to see if there was a relationship between complications after surgery and preoperative fitness levels [9]. In this study, 109 gastric bypass patients with morbid obesity (a BMI greater than 40 which generally coincides with being 100 pounds over ideal body weight) underwent VO2 fitness assessments preoperatively. (VO2 is defined as the maximum amount of oxygen that a person can take in and process during exercise). The mean age of patients in the study was 46, and the mean BMI was 48.7. VO2 peak values were measured preoperatively, and patients were placed in one of three VO2 categories:

- Group 1 = 13.7 mL/kg/min.
- Group 2 = 17.1 mL/kg/min.
- Group 3 = 21.2 mL/kg/min.

Understand that the higher one's VO2, the more fit the individual. Thus, the patients in group 3, who had the highest VO2 values, were considered to be in better shape than those in groups 1 and 2. After each patient underwent surgery, results suggested that poor cardiorespiratory fitness (measured by exercise testing) was a predictor of an increased risk of potentially fatal intraoperative and postoperative complications. Time in surgery for those in group 1 was longer, on average, by 24.8 minutes, compared with time in surgery for those in group 3. For patients in group 1, the length of hospital stay was one day longer, on average, and 30-day re-admission rates were highest for them (i.e., the patients with the lowest cardiorespiratory fitness). In addition, patients in group 1 were six times more likely to suffer surgery-related complications than those in the two other groups combined. It is important to note that the cardiorespiratory fitness levels for all three groups were considered poor to fair, compared to normative (good) fitness levels. This study underscores the importance of achieving a good-to-excellent level of cardiorespiratory fitness prior to undergoing bariatric surgery [9]. If you plan to have bariatric surgery, it is important to achieve an optimal level of fitness preoperatively and postoperatively. Refer to the following exercise guidelines for each stage of your surgery.

PREOPERATIVE STAGE

Do your best to get yourself prepared for surgery by improving your physical fitness as much as possible. The higher your level of fitness before surgery, the fewer complications you'll experience during and after surgery. The following general guidelines should prove helpful:

- Make weight loss a primary goal of your exercise program. Excess adipose tissue (fat) can make it much more difficult for your surgeon to find the

organs he/she is trying to operate on; it also can make the operation itself more challenging. In fact, your surgeon may even require that you lose a certain amount of weight before he/she will operate.
- Also focus on cardiovascular exercise to improve your heart health, decrease your body weight, and help you lose body fat before surgery.
- Follow the exercise guidelines discussed in the previous section of this chapter (Obesity in Adults).
- Follow your surgeon's recommendations for preoperative weight loss and all other exercise guidelines, depending on any other physical restrictions or limitations you may have.

POSTOPERATIVE STAGE

- If you have any postoperative complications—that is, physical problems following your weight-loss surgery—schedule an appointment with your bariatric surgeon and follow your surgeon's recommendations for an exercise program.
- For the first four weeks after surgery, focus on flexibility exercises, deep breathing, and getting back into performing your normal daily activities.
- Gradually incorporate low-intensity aerobic exercise (e.g., walking, biking, working out on an upper extremity bike).
- If your surgery was laparoscopic, it is generally safe to start exercising up to your pain threshold two weeks after surgery.
- If your surgery was incisional (open-cut) surgery, it may take a few more weeks to recover; therefore:
  1. During the first six weeks after surgery, do not lift any more than 15 lb; otherwise, exercise up to your pain threshold.
  2. Avoid abdominal exercises for the first eight to 12 weeks (i.e., allow the incision to fully heal). This will help alleviate abdominal hernias near or around the incision.
  3. Start exercising slowly and gradually progress.
  4. Significantly reduce your caloric intake. During the first few weeks to months after surgery, you should consume less than 500 calories a day, sometimes only 200-300 calories a day. (Your bariatric surgeon will give you specific instructions.) This significant decrease in calories may initially cause some fatigue. Therefore, you should not perform high-intensity exercise because you need to limit the number of carbohydrates you

metabolize (burn) since you are not consuming a large number of calories. Keep in mind that this is only during the initial postoperative stage. As you lose weight and increase your fitness level, you'll be able to take in a few more calories as well as exercise at higher levels of intensity. Again, follow your surgeon's dietary recommendations.

- Perform aerobic exercise at a low to moderate level of intensity. This is the most efficient way to decrease body fat safely after your surgery. The idea is to force your body to continue burning fat due to your limited intake of calories, remembering that your goal is to lose fat pounds. Realize that you can have a direct effect on losing fat by training your body to be maximally effective at burning fat. Refer to Chapter 7 for specifics on how to go about doing this.
- Your bariatric surgeon may increase your caloric intake to 1,200-1,400 calories six to 12 months after surgery, particularly if, at this point, you have lost a large percentage of your excess weight. Follow your surgeon's and/or dietician's recommendations on food intake.
- Follow the exercise guidelines described in the previous "Obesity in Adults" section of this chapter.
- Realize that if you have had weight-loss surgery, a lifelong exercise program is critical to your long-term success in maintaining a healthy weight and overall physical fitness. Bariatric surgery is a valuable tool for you to lose weight rapidly; however, in two to three years, if you have not adopted a physically active lifestyle, particularly a regular exercise program, you will start gaining the weight back. Throughout my years of working with bariatric surgery patients, I have personally witnessed some patients gain back large amounts of weight because they stopped or never started exercising. Exercising on a regular schedule is essentially the only thing that will help increase your metabolism and burn fat. Exercise becomes even more important postoperatively because the surgery itself, as well as your decreased intake of calories and rapid weight loss, dramatically lowers your metabolism and thus your body's fat-burning efficiency. According to an article in the *International Journal of Obesity*, a person's total energy expenditure can be significantly decreased as a result of a lowered metabolic rate following bariatric surgery [10]. You must combat this phenomenon through regular exercise. If you can stick to this advice, you'll be "cruising skinny" at a healthy weight and in good physical condition years after your surgery.

- Throughout your life, regularly monitor the progress you are making in your exercise program to ensure continued compliance with exercise that effectively controls your weight.

WHEELCHAIR BOUND OR AMPUTEE

If you are wheelchair bound, exercise should still be an important part of your day for flexibility, upper body strength, and cardiovascular fitness. It is especially important to have good flexibility as well as upper body strength in order to transfer easily and safely to and from your wheelchair.

WHEELCHAIR TRANSFER

Develop a safe method for easily transferring yourself to and from the wheelchair. If you have trouble transferring yourself, there are gait belts and/or transfer boards, which can make transferring much easier. In addition, you can seek training on proper transfer from a physical therapist (PT), occupational therapist (OT), or nurse. Your physician can write a prescription for rehabilitation and transfer training with a PT or OT.

If you are wheelchair bound, use the following steps to transfer yourself safely and as easily as possible to and from your wheelchair [11]:

1. Position the wheelchair parallel, yet at an angle, to the middle of the surface to which you are trying to transfer—that is, the wheelchair handle should be in the middle of the surface to which you are moving.
2. Lock the wheelchair.
3. Remove your feet from the foot rest and swing the foot rest out of the way.
4. Remove the wheelchair arm rest nearest the surface to which you are moving.
5. Move to the edge of the wheelchair so that you do not hit your bottom on the wheel nearest the surface to which you are moving when you slide from the wheelchair to the surface.
6. Place your hand on the closest surface of the location to which you are moving.
7. Use both arms to push up and lift your body off the seat of the chair. Be sure to keep your upper body erect, with your head positioned over the hips.
8. Scoot your body about 2-3 inches at a time until you are on the surface to which you are transferring.
9. Scoot yourself back and swing your legs around.

Understanding and Accepting Your Limitations: Exercising Without Injury

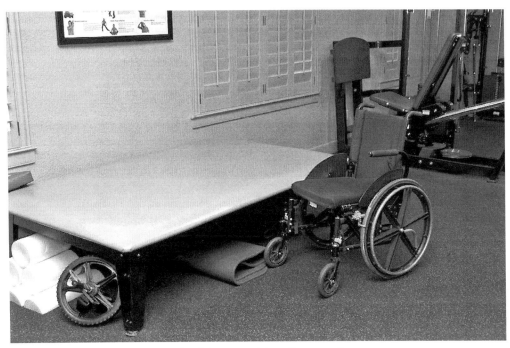

Wheelchair position for transfer.

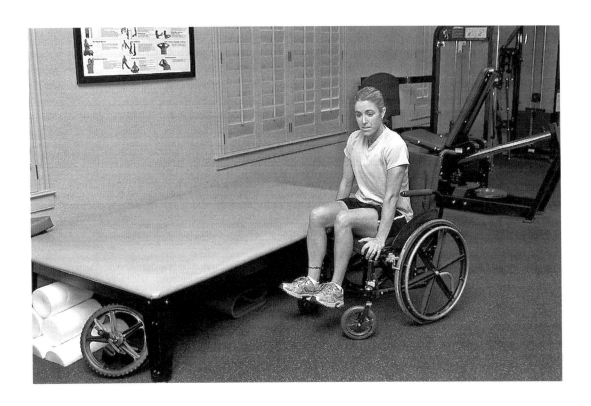

Rx Fitness for Weight Loss: The Medically Sound Solution to Get Fit and Save Your Life

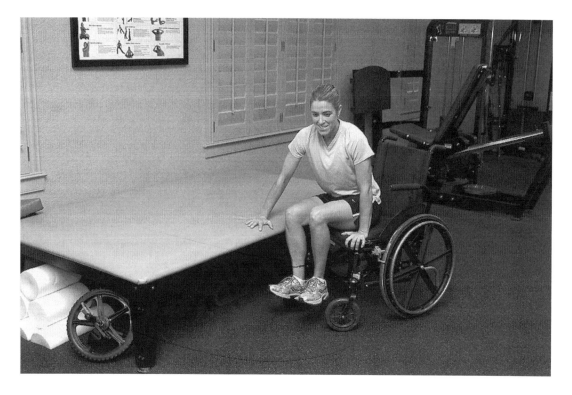

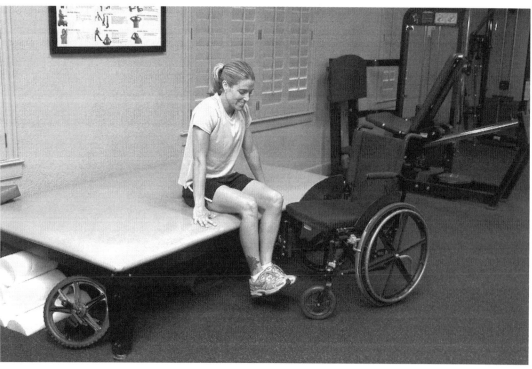

ROUTINE DAILY ACTIVITIES

Movement on a regular basis is very important to prevent atrophy of muscles, open sores, and decrease the risk of pneumonia and blood clots:

1. Frequently change the position of your hips. Do not sit in your chair for long periods of time; take 20-minute breaks and try to lie on your back or stomach two or three times a day.
2. If you have an amputated leg, do not hang your stump over the side of the bed and do not place a pillow under your stump unless otherwise told to do so by your physician or surgeon.
3. Stretch and move all joints through their entire range of motion daily; this will help maintain or even increase your joint mobility.

EXERCISE

Start slowly and gradually progress in your exercise regimen. Investment in a well-qualified fitness professional is highly recommended to help you achieve your fitness goals. Personal training can be of tremendous value for someone who is wheelchair bound because a trainer can help with the equipment setup as well as with demonstration of the exercises, guide your through your performance of them, and motivate you during your training sessions. Just make sure you are working with a professional trainer.

If you are wheelchair bound, you'll need to be actively involved in your rehabilitation and overall exercise program. Exercise is even more important for the wheelchair bound, since muscle atrophy (weakness from a decrease in muscle size) can occur quickly if the muscles are not being used on a regular basis. All four pillars of fitness (flexibility, cardio, strength, and healthy diet) should be followed in order to be physically fit and to maintain a healthy weight.

STRETCHING

For the wheelchair bound, the rules of thumb for stretching are not much different than those for other individuals:

1. Stretching should never be painful; hold a stretch only until you feel a light, yet comfortable pull.
2. Stretch on a daily basis and hold each stretch for at least 10-30 seconds.

3. Do not bounce while stretching; hold a stationary, or static, position. If your lower extremities are either nonexistent or severely limited with regard to overall strength or usability, you may need the assistance of another person to perform lower body stretches. Again, follow the general rules of thumb listed above. Use a flat stretch table or your bed to perform lower body stretches.

STRENGTH TRAINING

Many wheelchair-bound individuals still have use and strength of the upper body; however, it is common for them to experience neck and shoulder pain because they are constantly using the upper body to move themselves around. From using the arms to push their wheels, to transferring their body from a chair to a bed or another surface, they are in constant use of the upper body. This is why it is critical for the wheelchair bound to perform strengthening exercises, especially for the upper body. If the upper body muscles are strong, there is less strain on the shoulder, elbows, and spine. Since the lower extremities are not that functional, a majority of exercises must be performed in a seated position. Resistance bands or cable-driven strength machines are great pieces of equipment to start a strength training program. Since several of traditional strength training exercises may need to be modified, it is highly recommend that if you are wheelchair bound, you seek a qualified fitness professional or physical therapist for specific guidance on an individualized strength training program.

CARDIO TRAINING

If you do not have full use of your lower body, your upper body can be used for cardiovascular training. Some amputees have been able to use their prosthetics and even run or participate in competitive sports, so never doubt your potential capabilities. If you do need to rely on the upper body, things like upper extremity bikes and arm ergometers can be used for cardio exercise. Swimming may be another type of activity you can do to improve your aerobic capacity. However, you'll need a safe method of transfer to and from the pool.

REFERENCES

1. The Cooper Institute. Texas Youth Evaluation Program. Available at: www.window.state.tx/us/specialrpt/obesitycost/fitness_evaluation.pdf; accessed September 2, 2008.

2. *A Field Guide to Type 2 Diabetes: The Essential Resource from the Diabetes Experts: 2.* Alexandria, VA: American Diabetes Association, 2004.
3. *ACSM's Exercise Management for Persons with Chronic Diseases and Disabilities*, 2nd Ed. Indianapolis: American College of Sports Medicine, 2003.
4. *ACSM's Guidelines for Exercise Testing and Prescription*, 7th Ed. Indianapolis: American College of Sports Medicine, 2006. Pp 44, 58, 61, 66-67, 69, 70, 189-191, 298.
5. Facts of Life. Issue Briefings for Health Reporters, Vol 5, No 1, January 2000. Special Series: Collaborative Management and Chronic Conditions. Available at: www.cfah.org/factsoflife/vol5no1.cfm; accessed November 17, 2008.
6. *Clinical Guidelines on the Identification, Evaluation, and Treatment of Overweight and Obesity in Adults.* The Evidence Report: September (Appendix V). Washington, DC: National Institute of Health, 1987.
7. Westcott, Wayne L. Youth and strength training: why and how? Available at: www.fitnessandkids.com; accessed August 14, 2007.
8. Westcott, Wayne L. Will your kids be fit or fat? Available at: www.fitnessandkids.com; accessed August 14, 2007.
9. McCullough, P, Gallegher, M, Dejong, A, et al. Cardiorespiratory fitness and short-term complications after bariatric surgery. *The Cardiopulmonary and Critical Care Journal: CHEST* 2006;(August):130:517-525.
10. Germert, W, Westerterp, K, Acker, B, et al. Energy, substrate, and protein metabolism in morbid obesity before, during, and after massive weight loss. *International Journal of Obesity* 2000;24:711-718.
11. *Non-Weight Bearing Transfer from Wheelchair to Bed.* Columbus: Ohio State University Medical Center, Department of Orthopedics, 2002. Pp 1, 2.

Chapter 7
Maximizing Your Body's Fat-Burning Capacity

Athletes tend to push themselves 120 percent while exercising because their main objective is to jump higher, run faster, or become stronger. If your main objective is weight loss, you don't need to push yourself this hard. What you need to do is find an appropriate intensity that will maximize your body's ability to burn calories, specifically fat calories. For some of you, this may be a difficult concept to grasp because you've always had the "no pain, no gain" mindset. The reality of maximizing your weight loss is to work smarter, not harder. Yes it's true; you don't have to "kill" yourself in order to lose weight. In fact, your body is actually better at burning fat at low to moderate intensities of activity, especially if you're just starting to exercise. Although most athletes tend to be leaner, you'll be delighted to know that you don't have to train like an athlete to maximize your body's ability to burn fat and ultimately become leaner.

First, let me describe how your body uses fuel for activity and movement. Throughout the day, your body uses calories obtained through food for its fuel. Most of you understand that if you consume more food than your body uses as fuel, you'll ultimately gain weight, and if you consume less food than your body burns, you should ultimately lose weight. What you may not know is exactly what kind of food the body uses as fuel.

FUEL SOURCES

There are three different fuel sources, and your body generally uses two of them: fat and carbohydrates. Consider these as your primary fuel sources.

The third fuel source is protein. Protein is not an efficient fuel source; its main purpose is to build and repair tissue, not to provide fuel or energy. Protein is the main nutrient used in the formation of new body tissue and cells (e.g., wound repair, skin regeneration, muscle growth). This is why you hear about people (i.e., body builders) who ingest large amounts of protein to try to build muscle. Eating some protein is also very important for people trying to lose weight because they need to preserve their lean muscle through the weight-loss phase. Eating protein helps prevent the body from tapping into lean muscle mass for fuel. This is important because lean muscle helps stoke the metabolism or, in the case of body builders, grow muscle mass.

The other important points about protein are that it cannot exist without nitrogen, one of the key elements of protein, and that the body cannot store nitrogen and thus excretes excessive nitrogen, that is, protein we consume but do not need for cell, tissue, or muscle repair or creation. This is one of the reasons that most weight-loss diets consist of more protein and fewer carbohydrates. Essentially, these diets promote the body's preservation of lean muscle and/or excretion of surplus ingested protein, thus preventing its storage of excessive calories that would ultimately be metabolized into fat.

Okay, enough about protein. What about fat and carbohydrates? I mentioned that these are the fuels we need to burn in order to go about our daily lives. Let's start with fat, since it is really what most of you are concerned about. Fat is utilized both at rest and during activity. How you metabolize or burn fat at rest is most directly related to what you eat; your body will burn what you feed it. Again, the analogy of your body being like a car should help explain this concept. If you put premium unleaded fuel in your car, this is what it is going to burn. By the same token, if you put regular unleaded fuel in your car, it has no choice but to burn the regular unleaded. Your body works in a similar fashion. If you eat a diet rich in fat, it will burn a majority of its calories at rest from fat. Similarly if you eat breads, pastas, fruits, and vegetables, your body will burn a majority of carbohydrates at rest. Now, sometimes it doesn't always work out exactly this way because our bodies consist of tiny components called *genes*. I'm sure you realize that part of the reason you may be the way you are is because of your genetic makeup, or heredity (traits you inherited from your parents and other ancestors). In addition to the foods you consume, your genetic makeup also has a lot to do with the type of calories you burn in a resting state. In other words, some of us were simply born fat burners. Yes, we've all met these people. You know, the ones that can sit around the office and munch on donuts in the morning, eat out for lunch every day, enjoy a Snickers bar in the afternoon, and never gain a pound. You probably "hate" these people. And then others are just good carb burners: Their bodies "want" to burn carbohydrates and they hardly burn an ounce of fat at rest. You can "thank" your parents, grandparents, aunts, and uncles for these traits. If you're not a born fat burner, do not dismay because you can do a lot to combat some of those non-fat burning traits you've inherited.

One of the fastest ways to burn more fat at rest is to eat a well-balanced diet. If you eat a balanced diet consisting of the right amount of carbohydrates, fats, and protein; your body will burn about 60 percent of your calories from fat and about 40 percent from carbohydrates in a resting state [1]. That's not a bad ratio of fat burn simply from eating sensibly. Diets that are high in protein and low in carbohydrate will significantly help create an even better fat-burning body. These diets essentially force your body to burn fat because you're not consuming the easily digested carbohydrate and the body doesn't like to use protein for fuel. Thus, the body turns to the stored fat and begins to break it down for fuel. This process is called *ketosis*. The body breaks down fat to produce glucose and a byproduct called *ketones* to use for fuel. Refer to Chapter 4 for a description of the most advantageous dietary balance of fat, carbohydrates, and protein for weight loss and overall health.

You may be wondering what *at rest* means. It refers to a resting state as opposed to a physically active state. When you're exercising or physically active, your body burns fuel a bit differently. What type of calories you burn at rest has everything to do with your diet and genetics, whereas what type you burn while exercising has everything to do with your fitness level. Generally speaking, your body will burn fat or carbohydrate for fuel during exercise, as it does in a resting state, but your body will burn *fat* better at low to moderate workout intensities. The more intense your exercise, the more carbohydrates your body will burn. The reason for this is because it takes a lot longer to break down and metabolize or burn fat. Fat consists of long-chain fatty acids that are more difficult for the body to break down (metabolize). Unlike carbohydrate, fats (lipids) are insoluble in water; thus, digestion and absorption are more complicated. It all goes back to the Krebs cycle. Now I won't bore you with a detailed explanation of the Krebs cycle, but you need to understand that before the fat even enters the Krebs cycle, it must be broken down into free fatty acids and glycerol, which is broken down even further to acetyl CoA. This whole process takes some time, and therefore the body is more efficient at burning fat calories at lower intensities because the body doesn't need a whole lot of energy real quick. The bottom line is you'll burn a greater percentage of fat exercising at lower intensities. This is especially the case for those of you that are just starting an exercise regimen. This is great news for anyone trying to lose weight! Again, you don't have to "kill" yourself in order to lose fat pounds.

    Keep in mind that the body must utilize oxygen in order to burn fat. *Aerobic exercise* basically means exercise involving the intake of a considerable amount of oxygen. When you exercise aerobically, you are utilizing a large amount of oxygen to burn calories. Conversely, *anaerobic exercise* means exercising at a level at which oxygen debt occurs because the need for oxygen exceeds the capacity of the circulation to supply it. This generally occurs with short bursts of high-intensity exercise such as a 100-meter dash, vertical jumps, power lifts, or the explosiveness of a defensive lineman at the snap of a football. When the body is in an anaerobic state, it's only capable of burning carbohydrate. The best thing about this whole process is that you can actually make your body more efficient at burning fat at higher intensities and longer durations through training, and this should ultimately be everyone's goal. In other words, if you train your body the right way through exercise, it can become a better fat burner. If you are disciplined in training specifically to create the best fat-burning body possible, you'll inevitably have an easier time losing weight and ultimately be able to maintain a healthy weight once you've achieved your target weight. This helps explain why fit people tend to be leaner: They've created a body that is very good at burning fat and therefore it is easier for them to manage their weight.

    Before I tell you how to create an efficient fat-burning body, let me explain how your body uses carbohydrates for fuel. Carbohydrates (carbs) are the preferred fuel source to some degree. I say this because carbs are usually abundant in our bodies. The reason for this is because most people ingest a large number of carbs every day, and the body stores carbs in the liver and muscles. The stored carbs in your muscles is called *glycogen*. As you begin to move, your muscles can easily use this glycogen for energy. In addition to the carbs being stored in your muscles, your body prefers to utilize carbs because they are much easier to break down than the other two macronutrients: fat and protein. This also explains why your body will resort to burning more and more carbs when you exercise at higher intensities. More intense exercise requires quick energy, so the body resorts to burning carbs because it can get to them faster and break them down more quickly.

Great news, right? You're probably thinking yeah . . . yeah . . . but how do I do it? How do I exercise to create the most efficient fat-burning system? Do I just start moving? If so, for how long, how frequently, and how strenuously? Should I walk, bike, swim, or lift weights? These are all great questions.

Chapter 4 described the four pillars of fitness. One of the pillars, cardiovascular exercise, is the main support on which to lean for weight loss, specifically loss of fat pounds. The key is to know the point (exercise intensity) at which your body is most effective at burning fat. This is where heart-rate monitoring comes into play. Most of us have heard of people using a heart rate monitor while exercising. The reason you would want to do this is to ensure that you're training at the optimal intensity level to burn fat most efficiently. The point at which you are most effective at burning fat is considered to be your target heart rate, or aerobic base. It is the level of intensity, measured in beats per minute, at which your body can burn the most number of fat calories per minute. This is important to know if your main objective is fat loss. If you burn more fat calories while exercising, you'll have a better chance of losing the excess fat on your body. Now everyone is a bit different as to the point or exercise intensity that they are most efficient at burning fat; however, generally speaking most people are better at burning fat at low to moderate levels of exercise intensity. Not only will you burn more fat at lower intensities, but this will also be easier on your joints. In addition to promoting weight loss through burning more fat than carbs during exercise and preventing too much stress on your joints, a lower exercise intensity facilitates your body's adaptation to the new stress of exercise. This style of training also helps avoid overdoing exercise to a point at which you must temporarily suspend the exercise schedule you've set as your initial goal.

You might say, "Yes, but this goes against everything I've ever known or been told. I always thought you had to be huffing and puffing, or you weren't really doing any good." It is important to point out that there is a fine line here. The harder you work, the more total calories your body will burn. However, several problems come into play: Most of you won't be able to sustain this level of intensity for very long, and it is fairly hard on your joints if you haven't exercised consistently for some time. The other important consideration (and possible problem) is that you will be burning a greater percentage of carbs. You might be thinking "Well, a calorie is a calorie is a calorie, right?" Well, not exactly. Keep in mind that if you are combining your new exercise with a sensible diet that is generally low in carbs and high in lean protein (a very popular and effective diet for those trying to reduce their weight), you're really not consuming many carbs. So if you aren't eating many carbs and you have a whole lot of body fat to tap into, why would you want to burn more carbs through exercise? This would make it that much more difficult to stay on your diet after your workout. If you burn a bunch of carbs during exercise, after your workouts your body will tend to crave carbs, especially because you've been restricting them—not to mention that the fat you were trying to burn off during exercise is still hanging on, literally. This isn't what you want to accomplish. You can get yourself into a vicious and frustrating cycle by trying to exercise like this. The idea is to force your body to burn fat both through exercise *and diet*. If you're working hard in the gym, be sure you're burning and wasting away fat, not time.

Now, you're not going to train (exercise) at low intensities forever. Remember that your body reacts to how you train; thus, over time you'll have to work at higher levels to create a body that is good at burning fat at several different levels of intensity. In addition, you will reap more cardiovascular (heart health) benefits from exercising at higher levels and therefore you don't want to avoid it completely. The key is to prepare your body to be able to handle this level of stress. That is why you should start slowly and gradually progress in the intensity levels of your exercise program. Generally speaking, you'll want to increase the levels of your training every four to six weeks, provided you've been consistent with your previous exercise program. Eventually you'll want to progress in your levels of training so that you perform a variety of cardio intensities throughout the week. For example, once you've built up your stamina and overall fitness level (this may take several months), your weekly cardio sessions may look something like this: One session consisting of a 45-minute low-intensity walk; a second session involving 30 minutes of moderate intensity on the elliptical machine; and a third session consisting of treadmill interval training, with 2-3 minute bouts of high-intensity training.

VO2 MAX TESTING TO DETERMINE YOUR TARGET HEART RATE

Getting back to determining your target heart rate, VO2 max testing is the most accurate way to determine this. Check your local health clubs to see if any of them offer this metabolic testing, also known as *indirect calorimetry, maximum oxygen uptake,* or *O2 testing*. The reason this type of test is the most accurate is because it is individualized. In other words, this test will tell you how *your* body utilizes oxygen to metabolize fat and carbs for energy and will also determine *your* overall cardiovascular fitness level, or VO2 max. VO2 max is essentially the maximum volume of oxygen your body can take in during inhalation and utilize to help burn calories, specifically fat calories, for energy. During exercise, once your body begins to expire more carbon dioxide that the amount of oxygen it is able to inhale, you have reached your anaerobic threshold. At this point your body begins to burn 100 percent carbohydrate for fuel and is no longer burning fat. Most people cannot sustain this exercise intensity level very long.

A fitness professional needs to administer VO2 max testing, which is performed with the individual being tested wearing a mask or head device with a tube leading from the mouth to a gas analyzer. The analyzer is able to determine exactly how much oxygen is being utilized and how much carbon dioxide is being expired. Some forms of metabolic testing are able to determine exactly how many calories and what type of calorie you are burning in relation to your heart rate during exercise. With this form of metabolic testing, your target heart rate is determined. As previously explained, your target heart rate is the point at which your body burns the greatest number of fat calories per minute. If the machine doesn't tell you exactly what that value is, determine your heart rate when the respiratory quotient (RQ), or respiratory exchange ratio (RER), is 0.70. The RQ, or RER, value is the ratio between carbon dioxide produced and oxygen consumed. The RQ, or RER, value at which the body is burning 100 percent lipids or fat is considered to be 0.70, whereas the RQ, or RER value at which the body is burning 100 percent carbohydrates is considered to be 1.0 [2]. Thus, your target heart rate occurs when the RQ value equals 0.70, and your anaerobic threshold occurs when the RQ value equals 1.00. If you do not actually reach the exact heart rate equivalent to these RQ values during the assessment, the person administering the test should select the heart rate value closest to the RQ values (0.7 and 1.00) to determine both your target heart rate and anaerobic threshold.

After the mask/head device is appropriately fitted, you'll begin to exercise on a piece of cardio equipment (e.g., treadmill, bike, elliptical, arm cycle). The test administrator will gradually increase the intensity of the exercise and try to bring you to an anaerobic threshold. This is the point at which the body is no longer utilizing oxygen to burn calories. At this particular point, the body begins to burn only carbs for fuel. One's anaerobic threshold usually occurs at a fairly high intensity. This level of intensity should not initially be used to prescribe cardiovascular exercise for someone trying to lose weight. If you've completed VO2 metabolic testing, use the information below to calculate your three different training zones:

- *Fat-burning zone* = +/- five beats from the target heart rate, the point at which you burn the most amount of fat calories or the RQ value is equal or closest to 0.70. The range of this zone may be larger if you are in better shape and your body is able to burn fat for longer periods of time.
- *Fit zone* = 10-beats-per-minute zone that starts out 10-15 beats greater than the target heart rate
- *Threshold zone* = 10-beats-per-minute zone that falls close to or includes the anaerobic threshold

Example of training zones determined from metabolic testing:

- *Test results*
  1. VO2 max = 32.3 mL/kg/min
  2. Target heart rate = 124
  3. Anaerobic threshold = 163
- *Fat-burning zone* = 119-129 bpm
- *Fit zone* = 134-144 bpm
- *Threshold zone* = 154-164 bpm

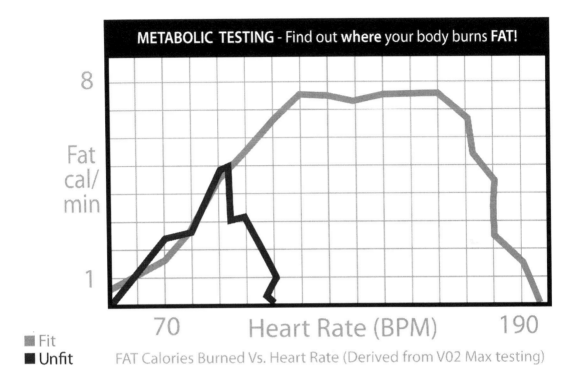

FAT Calories Burned Vs. Heart Rate (Derived from VO2 Max testing)

If you look at the fat calories burned versus heart rate chart derived from VO2 testing, you'll see that one can determine how many fat calories he/she burns according to his/her heart rate. In this particular example, the black line shows that this particular person's body burns fat most efficient at a heart rate of 93 beats per minute. Thus, if this individual wants to maximize the amount of fat burned while exercising, he/she would want to do cardiovascular exercise while keeping the heart rate at 93 beats per minute (bpm), or utilize a fat-burning zone ranging from 88-98 bpm. If you look at the gray line, this depicts an ideal assessment wherein the person has trained their body to be very efficient at burning fat. This person can essentially burn just as much fat at a heart rate of 120 bpm as they can a heart rate of 170 bpm. They also have a much higher anaerobic threshold than the person with the black-line test results.

If you are able to perform the metabolic test, record your results and training zones in the following chart.

Metabolic Test Results	Training Zones
VO2 max (mL/kg/min) _____	Fat-burning zone (bpm) _____
Target heart rate (bpm) _____	Fit zone (bpm) _____
Anaerobic threshold (bpm) _____	Threshold zone (bpm) _____

KARVONEN METHOD TO DETERMINE TARGET HEART RATE

Another method of determining your target heart rate or your fat-burning zone is to use an equation called the *Karvonen method*. This equation uses one's theoretical max heart rate (MHR) as well as resting heart rate (RHR) to determine different training zones. There is an important caveat, however: If you are currently taking a beta blocker or any other type of blood pressure medication that significantly lowers the heart rate, the Karvonen method should not be used to determine your target heart rate because the Karvonen method was developed to assess the healthy person who is not taking any medication that would lower his/her heart rate.

To apply the Karvonen method, you first need to determine both your max heart rate and your resting heart rate. Follow the simple instructions given in the next chapter under the heading "Heart Rate" to determine these values. Once you have these values, plug them (resting heart rate and maximum heart rate) into the equations below to determine your training zones. Once you've done this, record your values in the following Karvonen method results chart.

Karvonen Method Results

Fat-burning zone
(MHR − RHR) × 50% + RHR = _____
(MHR − RHR) × 60% + RHR = _____

Fit zone
(MHR − RHR) × 60% + RHR = _____
(MHR − RHR) × 70% + RHR = _____

Threshold zone
(MHR − RHR) × 70% + RHR = _____
(MHR − RHR) × 80% + RHR = _____

EXAMPLE OF TRAINING ZONE CALCULATIONS USING THE KARVONEN METHOD

A 35-year-old female whose resting heart rate (RHR) is 73 bpm and max heart rate (MHR) is 185 bpm:

- *Fat-burning zone*
(185 − 73) × 50% + 73 = 129 bpm
(185 − 73) × 60% + 73 = 140 bpm

- *Fit zone*
(185 − 73) × 60% + 73 = 140 bpm
(185 − 73) × 70% + 73 = 151 bpm

- *Threshold zone*
(185 − 73) × 70% + 73 = 151 bpm
(185 − 73) × 80% + 73 = 163 bpm

    It is important to understand that I have adapted the percentages above from what has generally been accepted for calculating similar training zones. Through my experience in working with overweight people, I've discovered that using 50-60 as the percentage in the Karvonen method to determine the fat-burning zone is an excellent starting place for most individuals. Occasionally, I've even used a training zone of 40-50 percent for the fat-burning zone for individuals who have an extremely low level of fitness. Beginning at these lower intensities tends to foster longer commitment, less burnout, fewer injuries, and greater weight loss initially. Three training zones are more than enough to get you started, but as you increase your fitness and your body's overall ability to burn fat during exercise, it may become necessary to calculate more training zones. The following chart can be used for this purpose.

Karvonen Method Results	Training Zones
Max heart rate (bpm) _____ Resting heart rate (bpm) _____	Fat-burning zone (bpm) _____ Fit zone (bpm) _____ Threshold zone (bpm) _____

One final way to calculate your training zones is to start doing some cardio activity while monitoring your heart rate. As you begin to exercise, pay attention to what your intensity levels are. Determine what your heart rate is in relationship to the rate of perceived exertion (RPE) or your overall intensity level. This will help determine your different training zones. Refer to the RPE scale in Appendix B and notice that at an RPE of 3-4 you sense your exertion as moderate to somewhat hard; in other words, you can carry on a conversation but need to catch your breath occasionally. Identify what your heart rate is when you experience this type of intensity level of exertion. This heart rate will be your estimated target heart rate. Again, understand that this level of intensity is the best starting point for someone that's overweight or obese or simply not in good cardiovascular shape. Once you've identified this value, fill in your training zones in the following chart.

RPE to Heart Rate Method Results	Training Zones
Estimated target heart rate RPE 3-4 = _____ heart rate (bpm) Resting heart rate (bpm) _____	Fat-burning zone (bpm) _____ (+/- 5 beats around target heart rate) Fit zone (bpm) _____ (10-beat zone that starts 10-15 beats higher than target heart rate) Threshold zone (bpm) _____ (10-beat zone that starts 10-15 beats higher than highest fit-zone heart rate)

REFERENCES

1. Williams, Melvin H. *Nutrition for Health, Fitness, and Sport*, 6th Ed. New York: McGraw-Hill, 2002. P 91.
2. McArdle, W, Katch, F, and Katch, V. *Exercise Physiology: Energy, Nutrition, and Human Performance*, 4th Ed. Baltimore: Williams & Wilkins, 1996. Pp 145, 146.

Chapter 8
Performing Fitness Assessments and Reassessments

Part of the reason people become frustrated with their exercise program is because they claim they can't see any results. This underscores the importance of regular fitness assessments. You must be assessed and reassessed in order to truly know *if* you are making progress and *how much* progress you've made. Not only will you be able to understand your progress along the way, but you will also know where you stand as far as how physically fit you really are. Assessments will help you design your exercise program because you will identify areas in which you are strong as well as those in which you are weak. Often, people start off way too aggressively and end up getting hurt or sick because they don't understand their current fitness levels. This often leads to noncompliance with their exercise regimen.

You need to understand what type of assessments you should have, how frequently you should have them, and how to interpret the results of these assessments. This information can help you meet and surpass your wellness and weight loss goals. You'll know where you're at, where you need to go, and how you are doing along the way. So what type of assessments should you perform? Well, recall the main points in Chapter 4, which described the four pillars of fitness: flexibility, cardio, strength, and a healthy diet. Let's begin there. Now that you understand each pillar, or category, of fitness and why each is important to your overall success, you need to know how you rate for each category of fitness.

Keep in mind that the best way to accomplish fitness assessments is to have a professional fitness expert perform them. However, several assessments can be completed on your own or with the assistance of another individual. These types of assessments are often referred to as *field tests*, and this chapter outlines how to perform several different field tests. I also recommend that everyone have comprehensive lab work done initially and then every three to six months, depending on what your physician recommends. As you go through these assessments, be sure to accomplish each overall health-related assessment; then you can either accomplish all individual assessments or, at a minimum, accomplish one for each pillar of fitness. In other words, perform all health-related assessments as well as at least one flexibility assessment, one cardiovascular assessment, and one strength assessment.

OVERALL HEALTH-RELATED ASSESSMENTS

BLOOD PRESSURE

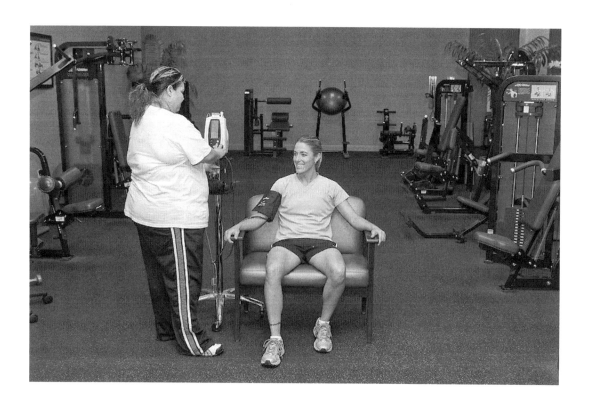

Blood pressure and heart rate assessments help reveal the condition of your heart, that is, your heart health. You can measure your blood pressure by yourself with a home device or have it measured at your physician's office. You may even want to explore the various health expos or health fairs in your area; they often offer different health screenings such as blood pressure for free. You can check your local newspaper to find out when and where these health screenings are to be held.

If you are taking your blood pressure with a home device, be sure to be seated quietly for at least 5 minutes before taking your blood pressure. There are several different blood pressure devices; the most common is used by wrapping it around the upper arm. Be sure to follow the instructions that come with your device, since closely following the outlined technique helps ensure the accuracy of blood pressure measurements. In addition to following the device's operating instructions, I advise that you take two or three readings on consecutive days at different times of the day. This will ensure an accurate reading under different circumstances (i.e., different times of the day).

Here are some basic instructions for most manual-inflation blood pressure monitors:

Sit down so that your feet are flat on the floor and your back is supported. Place the blood pressure cuff around your left arm; the bottom of the cuff should be about ½ inch above the elbow. The cuff tab or inflation hose of the device should lie over the brachial artery or the middle of the bicep (inside portion of the upper arm). Secure the cuff firmly around the arm and then relax the arm on a table, with the palm facing up. (Note that if the cuff is too tight or too small, it can skew pressure readings. Larger cuffs can be purchased if necessary). Turn the monitor on, and when prompted by the device, inflate the cuff to approximately 180 mm Hg. Keep still, and the device will automatically measure and display your blood pressure.

Record your blood pressure:_____ mm Hg

Understand that the blood pressure reading will display two numbers. The number you see displayed on the top is your systolic blood pressure score, and the number on the bottom is your diastolic reading. If either number is outside of the suggested ranges, you are considered to be prehypertensive or hypertensive. Refer to the following table to see in which classification your blood pressure (BP) falls: normal, prehypertensive, or hypertension.

Blood Pressure Classifications

Classification	Systolic BP mm Hg		Diastolic BP mm Hg
Normal	< 120	and	< 80
Prehypertension	120-139	or	80-89
Hypertension	≥ 140	or	≥ 90

Source: Modified from *ACSM's Guidelines for Exercise Testing and Prescription* [1].

If your blood pressure falls within the range for either the prehypertension or hypertension category, be sure to notify your physician and discuss treatment options. Generally, one of the first things your physician will do is prescribe lifestyle modifications. Unless your physician specifies otherwise, physical activity should be included in these modification recommendations. Refer to the hypertension section in Chapter 6 for specific exercise guidelines.

HEART RATE

Your heart rate is also an indicator of your physical health. The heart rate is measured in beats per minute (bpm), or the number of times the heart beats in 1 minute. The best way to measure your heart rate is to use a heart rate monitor. I recommend that anyone who is serious about losing weight purchase a heart rate monitor. Not only is it a good tool to use for heart rate assessments, but it also is extremely useful in making sure you train in a way that maximizes your body's fat-burning capacity. Refer to Chapter 7 for more information about how to maximize your body's ability to burn fat. Understand that the technique for heart rate assessments outlined below can be performed without a heart rate monitor (i.e., monitor for taking your pulse), but the results will not be quite as accurate. There are three different heart rate assessments you should perform: (1) resting heart rate *or* ambient heart rate, (2) maximum heart rate, and (3) recovery heart rate.

Performing Fitness Assessments and Reassessments

RESTING HEART RATE

This is your heart rate for 1 minute in a resting state. One is considered to be in a true resting state when lying down, so the best time to perform this assessment is first thing in the morning, preferably before you even get out of bed. Put your heart rate monitor on, but be sure to wet the sensors with water before placing around your chest. Once the monitor is on, be sure the chest strap is secure and working correctly. Relax and remain calm for 2-5 minutes before you record your heart rate. If you don't have a heart rate monitor, you should find your pulse with two fingers (index and middle fingers); do *not* use your thumb, since it also has a prominent pulse and may skew your heart rate reading. You can find your pulse either in your neck, at the carotid artery (just to the right of your Adam's apple), or in your wrist, at the radial artery (outside portion of the wrist, with the palm up).

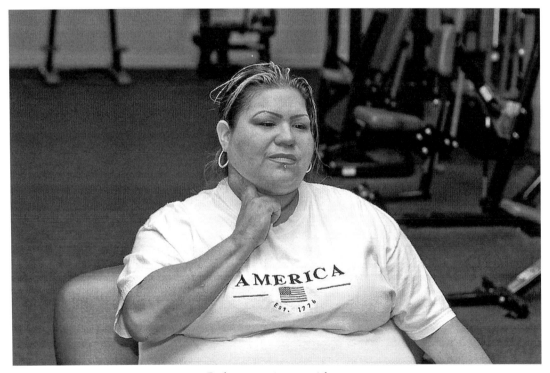

Pulse rate via carotid artery.

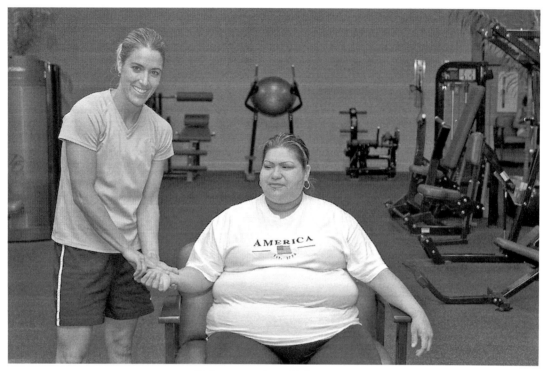
Pulse rate via radial artery.

Once you can feel your pulse, count the beats for a total of 30 seconds. Multiply this number by 2, and you will have your 1-minute resting heart rate in beats per minute (bpm). Your resting heart rate is a good indicator of your overall cardiovascular health. In general, a resting heart rate less than 80 bpm is pretty good; a rate between 60 and 70 bpm is even better. Your heart rate should decrease as you become more fit. If you notice that your resting heart rate becomes elevated for a few days in a row, you may be overtraining, or you may be ill or under a lot of stress.

Record your resting heart rate:_____ bpm

AMBIENT HEART RATE

This is your heart rate for 1 minute in a seated position, and measuring it is an alternative to measuring your resting heart rate. You measure your ambient heart rate in a manner similar to how you measure your resting heart rate. The only difference is that the measurement isn't done first thing in the morning and is performed while you are in a seated position—for example, sitting at your desk or watching television.

Record your ambient heart rate:_____ bpm

MAXIMUM HEART RATE

The maximum heart rate can be measured a couple of different ways. One method requires no exertion and is derived from an equation. This equation suggests that one's theoretic maximal heart rate is 220 minus his/her age. Keep in mind that using this equation is obsolete if you are taking a beta blocker because the medication significantly lowers the heart rate. Do not use this equation to determine max heart rate if you are taking a beta blocker.

Another, more accurate method to determine the maximum heart rate requires considerable exertion. This method can be used regardless of whether or not you're taking a beta blocker, but due to the high level of exertion required with this form of maximal heart rate testing, make sure your physician has cleared you to exercise with no limitations. Not including your warm-up and cool down, this test takes about 3-5 minutes to complete.

After you have properly warmed up, choose a form of cardiovascular activity that accommodates your physical state. Your warm-up should mirror the activity you've chosen to perform this test. Start to exercise and try to increase your heart rate by about 5 beats every 15-20 seconds. Keep doing this until you've reached your maximum level of exertion. At the point of your maximum effort—that is, the point at which you can't continue any longer or increase your heart rate any more—look to see what your heart rate value is and record this number. This is your maximum heart rate.

Record your maximum heart rate:_____ bpm

RECOVERY HEART RATE

This value will determine how efficient your heart is at recovering to a pre-exercising heart rate after maximizing your heart rate. Choose one of the following activities to perform this assessment: jumping jacks, jogging in place, stationary bike, climbing stairs, or punching with 2- to 5-lb dumbbells. The activity you choose should not aggravate any of your exercise restrictions/limitations—for example, if you have knee or spine complications, you should not have chosen jumping jacks. Once you've identified a form of exercise that works for you, perform your activity for 2 minutes at a quick and steady pace. Pick up your pace the last 30 seconds in an effort to maximize your heart rate and then record your heart rate immediately after the 2 minutes are up. Next, record your heart rate at the following intervals: 1 minute after stopping, 2 minutes after stopping, and 3 minutes after stopping. Do not sit down after you've stopped the exercise activity. You should be able to remain standing for the entire 3 minutes after you stop. As you get in better shape, your heart rate will "recover" at a quicker rate. In other words your 1-, 2-, and 3-minute recovery intervals will become lower values as you become more fit.

RECORD YOUR RECOVERY HEART RATES:

1-minute recovery heart rate:_____ bpm
2-minute recovery heart rate:_____ bpm
3-minute recovery heart rate:_____ bpm

POSTURE AND BALANCE ASSESSMENTS

POSTURE

Posture is very important, especially since it greatly affects one's physical activity. If you do not have good posture, you can easily injure yourself during exercise and cause further postural deviations.

I'm sure you've heard people say "Stand up straight," "Watch your posture," or "Stop slouching," or "Stop slumping." Many of us may think we know what good posture is, but few of us make a conscious effort to ensure our spines are supported by maintaining good posture.

Good posture involves training your body to maintain neutral alignment or stand, sit, walk, and lie in positions that cause the least amount of strain on your joints and muscles. Neutral alignment is basically standing with the feet about shoulder width apart, the back straight, the shoulders back, the chest out, and the chin parallel to the floor (see the figure in neutral alignment on the following page).

Before reading any further, perform the following posture evaluation. You can perform it alone, using a mirror, or another person can help you. This assessment is best evaluated while you're wearing minimal clothing; as your clothing may obstruct the ability to see any posture deviations. Answer the following questions and identify where your posture deviates from neutral alignment. Place check marks in the appropriate box next to what you see in the mirror or what the person helping to evaluate you notices about your posture:

1. Stand facing a mirror and identify the following:
   - *Head placement*: Is your head straight up and down and looking straight ahead? Or is your head slightly tilting to one side or the other.
     ☐ Straight up and down   ☐ Tilted to the righ   ☐ Tilted to the left

   - *Shoulder alignment:* As you look in the mirror, are your shoulders level from the right side to the left side, or do you see slight depression or elevation on one side over the other?
     ☐ Level from right to left   ☐ Right shoulder lower   ☐ Left shoulder lower

   - *Feet placement:* Are your feet close together, shoulder-width apart, or do you have a wide stance (feet more than shoulder-width apart).
     ☐ Shoulder width apart   ☐ Close together   ☐ Wide apart

2. Stand with a side profile to the mirror and identify the following:
   - *Head placement:* Is your chin pronated (jutting) forward? Is your chin level/parallel to the floor?
     ☐ Level/parallel to the floor   ☐ Pronated or jutting forward

   - *Shoulder alignment:* Are your shoulders rotated forward? Is the shoulder in line with the hips, knees, and ankles?
     ☐ Shoulders up and back   ☐ Rotated forward

   - *Lower body alignment:* Are your hips, knees, and ankles in alignment with one another?
     ☐ Hips over knees and knees over ankles   ☐ Hips tilted forward with knees bowed back

   - *Hips and core alignment:* Do you have an anterior pelvic tilt? In other words, is the upper portion of your pelvic girdle or hip bone rotated forward?
     ☐ Anterior pelvic tilt   ☐ Neutral alignment of hips over the knees

- *Back alignment:* Do you have excess curvature of either the cervical (kyphosis) or lumbar back (lordosis)? Is your spine straight, or do you have a sideways curvature (scoliosis)?

  ☐ Neutral/natural curvature ☐ Kyphosis ☐ Lordosis ☐ Scoliosis

Now that you've identified different items about your posture, please refer to the photographs below to see which you have: good or poor posture. Notice the items that contribute to poor posture and what is required for good posture.

GOOD POSTURE

Neutral alignment
Involves keeping your feet about shoulder width apart, with the toes pointing forward, shoulders back, chest out, and head up, with the chin in and parallel to the floor. Your hips, knees, and ankles should all fall in alignment with one another.

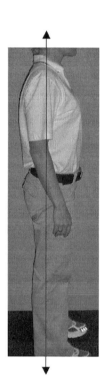

POOR POSTURE

Posture deviations:
- Forward rotation of the shoulders
- Anterior pelvic tilt - forward rotation of the hips or pelvic girdle
- Wide stance, with toes pointing out
- Head pronated forward
- Lordosis, or exaggerated curvature, of the lumbar spine
- Kyphosis, or exaggerated curvature, of the cervical spine
- Scoliosis, or sideways curvature, of the thoracic spine

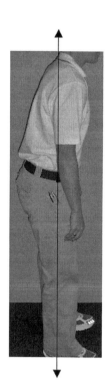

REQUIREMENTS FOR GOOD POSTURE
- Good flexibility and full joint range of motion
- Strong core muscles and other posture muscles, such as the upper back and legs
- A balance of muscular strength on each side of the body
- Conscious awareness and correction of your posture

FACTORS CONTRIBUTING TO POOR POSTURE
- Being overweight or obese
- Muscle imbalances due to weak muscles or poor flexibility
- Wearing high heels
- Poor work environment
- Improper lifting techniques
- Carrying a heavy bag or purse

BALANCE

We all need balance in our lives. If you think about it, every day of our lives is a balancing act. We are constantly balancing work, family, spiritual, emotional, physical, and personal needs. In order to accomplish all of this, we must have good balance. And no, I'm not just referring to your ability to decide which is more important or what needs to be accomplished first. Rather, I'm referring to your overall muscular strength and physical equilibrium, which helps keep everything moving ahead in the right direction. The inner ear balance system works with the eye's, muscles, and joints to maintain orientation or balance [2]. Thus, balance can greatly affect one's ability to perform daily activities. You might think there is no correlation, but in actuality there is a strong correlation. If your balance is poor, you could easily stumble and injure yourself. If you are injured, you will have great difficulty balancing all of the things listed above, and you definitely won't be able to maintain your new physically active regimen.

How do you know if your balance is good? Perform the assessment below and answer the questions:

1. Begin in a seated position and stand up. Sit back down. Did you have to use your hands or some other object to help you stand and/or sit? If so, this is an indication that you probably need to work on your balance.

2. From a standing position, shut your eyes for about 10-30 seconds. Did you notice any swaying? If so, this is an indication that you probably need to work on your balance.

3. From a standing position, slowly turn around in a 360-degree circle. Stop and do the same thing in the opposite direction. Were you able to take continuous steps or

did you have to stop, gather yourself, and take another step? If your steps weren't continuous, this is an indication that you probably need to work on your balance.

4. Look at your feet. Are they close together or fairly wide apart? If your feet are greater than 8 inches apart, this is an indication that you probably need to work on your balance.

Understand that there are different balance disorders. However, if you are overweight or obese, you may have struggled with the various actions listed in the above assessment due to the excess weight you are carrying around. For example, if you had to use your hands or another object to help yourself get up and down from the chair, it probably has to do with the fact that you have to lift a lot more weight than someone who is of normal size. In addition, you may have some limitation such as knee or back pain that you are trying to accommodate as you lift yourself in and out of a chair. Similarly, if you have discontinuous footsteps or a wide stance, this is more than likely due to your excess weight because, as you shift the weight around, it takes more effort to regain your balance. Think of it in terms of physics. Once you get an object moving, momentum takes over. The heavier the object, the more difficult it is to stop moving. If you're overweight, you have a lot more to support or hold up; therefore, you may need to gather yourself before attempting to take another step and/or you may need a wide stance to support all of your excess weight. Another issue to consider is that balance becomes more and more important as we age. According to Richard Boyle, "Falls among the elderly are a leading cause of debilitating injury (such as hip fractures) and a serious risk factor for premature death" [2]. This being said, if you lose some weight and increase your muscular strength, you will undoubtedly improve your balance and reduce your risk of injury.

BODY WEIGHT, BODY MASS INDEX, AND BODY COMPOSITION

WEIGHT

Measuring your body weight is fairly self-explanatory, but unfortunately many people tend to get obsessed with numbers on the scale, which often proves to be counterproductive. First and foremost, do not weigh yourself every day! I recommend that you weigh once a week. When you weigh, it is important to weigh yourself at relatively the same time of the day, wearing the same type of clothing or no clothing at all. This will help with consistency in your weight measurements. Remember that your weight is one of many assessments throughout your weight-loss journey. Don't get upset if the number on the scale isn't going down as fast as you'd like. While you may not initially be losing weight, you may be losing inches, lowering your blood pressure, improving your strength, etc. The weight *will* come off; you just have to be persistent and stay consistent. Remember that fitness is the secret to long-term weight management, but there are many other pieces to the puzzle, such as dietary intake, emotional and spiritual well-being, and medical conditions.

Record your weight here:_____ lb

HEIGHT

Now that you know your weight, you also need to know your height. It is always a good idea to measure your height even though you think you know how tall you are. Sometimes you aren't as tall as you once were; as we age our bodies change in posture, bone density, joint padding, and muscular mass, all of which can affect height.

Record your height here:_____ inches

BODY MASS INDEX

If you know your height and weight, you can determine your body mass index (BMI) by referring to the following table or calculating it using this equation:

$$BMI = \text{weight (lb)} \div [\text{height (in)}]^2 \times 703$$

Record your BMI here:_____

Body Mass Index (BMI) Values Based on Height and Weight

BMI	19	20	21	22	23	24	25	26	27	28	29	30	31	32	33	34	35
Height (inches)						Body Weight (lb)											
58	91	96	100	105	110	115	119	124	129	134	138	143	148	153	158	162	167
59	94	99	104	109	114	119	124	128	133	138	143	148	153	158	163	168	173
60	97	102	107	112	118	123	128	133	138	143	148	153	158	163	168	174	179
61	100	106	111	116	122	127	132	137	143	148	153	158	164	169	174	180	185
62	104	109	115	120	126	131	136	142	147	153	158	164	169	175	180	186	191
63	107	113	118	124	130	135	141	146	152	158	163	169	175	180	186	191	197
64	110	116	122	128	134	140	145	151	157	163	169	174	180	186	192	197	204
65	114	120	126	132	138	144	150	156	162	168	174	180	186	192	198	204	210
66	118	124	130	136	142	148	155	161	167	173	179	186	192	198	204	210	216
67	121	127	134	140	146	153	159	166	172	178	185	191	198	204	211	217	223
68	125	131	138	144	151	158	164	171	177	184	190	197	203	210	216	223	230
69	128	135	142	149	155	162	169	176	182	189	196	203	209	216	223	230	236
70	132	139	146	153	160	167	174	181	188	195	202	209	216	222	229	236	243
71	136	143	150	157	165	172	179	186	193	200	208	215	222	229	236	243	250
72	140	147	154	162	169	177	184	191	199	206	213	221	228	235	242	250	258
73	144	151	159	166	174	182	189	197	204	212	219	227	235	242	250	257	265
74	148	155	163	171	179	186	194	202	210	218	225	233	241	249	256	264	272
75	152	160	168	176	184	192	200	208	216	224	232	240	248	256	264	272	279
76	156	164	172	180	189	197	205	213	221	230	238	246	254	263	271	279	287

BMI	36	37	38	39	40	41	42	43	44	45	46	47	48	49	50	51	52	53	54
Height (inches)						Body Weight (lb)													
58	172	177	181	186	191	196	201	205	210	215	220	224	229	234	239	244	248	253	258
59	178	183	188	193	198	203	208	212	217	222	227	232	237	242	247	252	257	262	267
60	184	189	194	199	204	209	215	220	225	230	235	240	245	250	255	261	266	271	276
61	190	195	201	206	211	217	222	227	232	238	243	248	254	259	264	269	275	280	285
62	196	202	207	213	218	224	229	235	240	246	251	256	262	267	273	278	284	289	295
63	203	208	214	220	225	231	237	242	248	254	259	265	270	278	282	287	293	299	304
64	209	215	221	227	232	238	244	250	256	262	267	273	279	285	291	296	302	308	314
65	216	222	228	234	240	246	252	258	264	270	276	282	288	294	300	306	312	318	324
66	223	229	235	241	247	253	260	266	272	278	284	291	297	303	309	315	322	328	334
67	230	236	242	249	255	261	268	274	280	287	293	299	306	312	319	325	331	338	344
68	236	243	249	256	262	269	276	282	289	295	302	308	315	322	328	335	341	348	354
69	243	250	257	263	270	277	284	291	297	304	311	318	324	331	338	345	351	358	365
70	250	257	264	271	278	285	292	299	306	313	320	327	334	341	348	355	362	369	376
71	257	265	272	279	286	293	301	308	315	322	329	338	343	351	358	365	372	379	386
72	265	272	279	287	294	302	309	316	324	331	338	346	353	361	368	375	383	390	397
73	272	280	288	295	302	310	318	325	333	340	348	355	363	371	378	386	393	401	408
74	280	287	295	303	311	319	326	334	342	350	358	365	373	381	389	396	404	412	420
75	287	295	303	311	319	327	335	343	351	359	367	375	383	391	399	407	415	423	431
76	295	304	312	320	328	336	344	353	361	369	377	385	394	402	410	418	426	435	443

Source: Adapted from *Clinical Guidelines on the Identification, Evaluation, and Treatment of Overweight and Obesity in Adults. The Evidence Report: September* [3].

Now that you have determined your BMI, refer to the following table of BMI ranges relative to weight status to determine your weight status.

BMI	Weight Status
Below 18.5	Underweight
18.5-24.9	Normal
25.0-29.9	Overweight
30.0-34.9	Obesity class I
35.0-39.9	Obesity class II
Greater than or equal to 40.0	Obesity class III

Source: Adapted from *ACSM's Guidelines for Exercise Testing and Prescription* [1].

BODY COMPOSITION

Body composition is a more comprehensive measurement than BMI. Your BMI may place you in a weight classification (i.e., underweight, normal, overweight, or obese), but it doesn't determine your body fat or fat-free mass. Thus, you could actually be in the overweight or obese range despite falling within a normative body-fat range. This is often the case for some athletes and body builders.

Body fat is often thought of as being negative or really bad. However, we actually need a certain amount of body fat for our bodies to function on a daily basis. Body fat helps cushion our joints and protect our organs. It also helps regulate body temperature, facilitates absorption and utilization of vitamins, and helps the body sustain itself when food is scarce. Problems occur when we have too much or too little fat and the excess or lack thereof begins to affect our bodies negatively, which in turn causes serious health risks.

There are several methods to test for body composition; a relatively easy and inexpensive method is bioelectrical impedance. Currently there are several types of home scales that measure weight *and* body-fat percentage using bioelectrical impedance, but if you do not have access to this equipment, search for local wellness centers and give them a call to see if they perform body-fat percentage tests.

Another method of body-fat testing is through the use of calipers, a pliers or tong-like tool that "grabs" body fat to measure it. This method is difficult to perform with accuracy on people who are overweight due to their excess adipose tissue: It is challenging to pinch the accurate amount of body fat; often, too much or too little tissue is grabbed, or pinched. Hydrostatic weighing is considered to be the gold standard, but it is also fairly cumbersome to perform. This method of body fat testing would have to be performed in a wellness or athletic facility.

Whichever method you choose to use, just remember to be consistent and use the same method for reassessment so you accurately measure your improvement and effectively track your progress. Depending on which method used to determine your body composition, you should obtain one or more of the following data: body fat, fat-free mass, and total water weight.

BODY FAT

See normative ranges for body-fat percentage measurements for men and women in the following tables.

Body Composition (% Body Fat) for Men

Percentile	Age				
	20-29	30-39	40-49	50-59	60+
90 Well above average	7.1	11.3	13.6	15.3	15.3
80	9.4	13.9	16.3	17.9	18.4
70 Above average	11.8	15.9	18.1	19.8	20.3
60	14.1	17.5	19.6	21.3	22.0
50 Average	15.9	19.0	21.1	22.7	23.5
40	17.4	20.5	22.5	24.1	25.0
30 Below average	19.5	22.3	24.1	25.7	26.7
20	22.4	24.2	26.1	27.5	28.5
10 Well below average	25.9	27.3	28.9	30.3	31.2

Source: Adapted from *ACSM's Guidelines for Exercise Testing and Prescription* [1].

Body Composition (% Body Fat) for Women

Percentile	Age				
	20-29	30-39	40-49	50-59	60+
90 Well above average	14.5	15.5	18.5	21.6	21.1
80	17.1	18.0	21.3	25.0	25.1
70 Above average	19.0	20.0	23.5	26.6	27.5
60	20.6	21.6	24.9	28.5	29.3
50 Average	22.1	23.1	26.4	30.1	30.9
40	23.7	24.9	28.1	31.6	32.5
30 Below average	25.4	27.0	30.1	33.5	34.3
20	27.7	29.3	32.1	35.6	36.6
10 Well below average	32.1	32.8	35.0	37.9	39.3

Source: Adapted from *ACSM's Guidelines for Exercise Testing and Prescription* [1].

According to Health Check Systems, The American Council on Exercise has categorized ranges of body-fat test percentages as shown in the following table.

Body-Fat Test Percentages

Description	Women	Men
Essential fat	12-15%	2-5%
Athletes	16-20%	6-13%
Fitness	21-24%	14-17%
Acceptable	25-31%	18-25%
Obese	32%+	25%+

Most bioelectrical impedance body-composition devices will give you total fat-free mass and total body water.

FAT-FREE MASS

Fat-free mass is your weight, excluding body fat. It includes the weight of bone, muscle tissue, and water. It is important to keep track and be aware of what your fat-free mass is before you start an exercise or weight-loss program. Your main goal is to maintain your fat-free mass through the weight-loss phase. Often, if you begin to reduce your caloric intake too much or too quickly in an effort to lose weight, your body will start to metabolize muscle for fuel to use as its energy source. Since energy isn't readily available due to the caloric restriction, your body may tap into lean muscle and use it for energy. This is especially true for individuals who experience rapid weight loss, such as someone who has had weight-loss surgery. One doesn't want to lose any lean muscle mass because retaining lean muscle tissue helps keep your metabolism working efficiently. The more lean muscle you have the more calories it takes to sustain that muscle. It takes more energy to sustain lean muscle mass vs. fat mass. Thus, your goal is to lose fat and keep the muscle. You can help minimize loss of fat-free mass through a regular weight or strength training program.

TOTAL BODY WATER

Total body water is the amount of water in your body. Believe it or not, our bodies consist of a lot of water. In fact, the water in your body can constitute anywhere from 40 percent to 75 percent of your total body weight. The reason for the large disparity is because the percentage of water in your body has a lot to do with how much adipose tissue, or fat, your body contains. Adipose tissue contains less than 10 percent water; muscle, on the other hand, contains nearly 70 percent water. Thus, it is important that you avoid becoming dehydrated during exercise. See the following normative ranges for total body water [4]:

- Healthy ranges for men = 50-65 percent
- Healthy ranges for women = 45-60 percent

GIRTH MEASUREMENTS

A pound of muscle weighs the same as a pound of fat. A pound is a pound is a pound. Many people believe that muscle weighs more than fat, but this is not exactly true. If you put a pound of muscle on a scale and a pound of fat on a scale, they will both weigh exactly the same: 1 lb. The difference is in the diameter of each pound. A pound of muscle is leaner and thus smaller in diameter than a pound of fat. Muscle is more dense than fat. This is why you can lose inches but not lose weight. This is also why it is important to take girth measurements before you start your exercise program and throughout it—to identify how many total inches you've lost. If I had to choose between inches and weight, I would pick inches every time. Why? Well, if I am smaller in inches, it means my clothes fit better, which probably makes me feel and look better. Again, this is why I discourage people from weighing themselves every day. So, what measurements should you be taking? The more measurements you take, the more you will know. Body circumference measurements are referred to as *girth measurements*. Basically, when you perform girth measurements, you measure the distance, or girth, around different areas of your body. You should use a plastic or Gulick tape measuring device to take these measurements. As you perform and record each measurement listed in the following chart, keep your muscles relaxed and don't "squish" yourself.

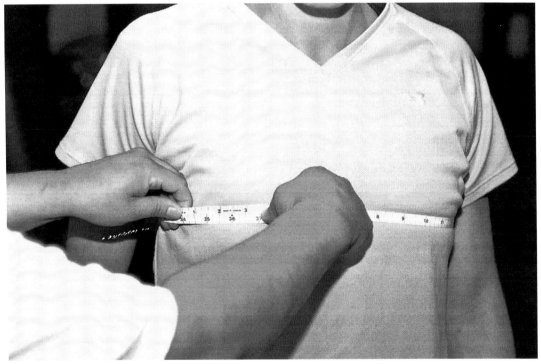

Chest girth measurement.

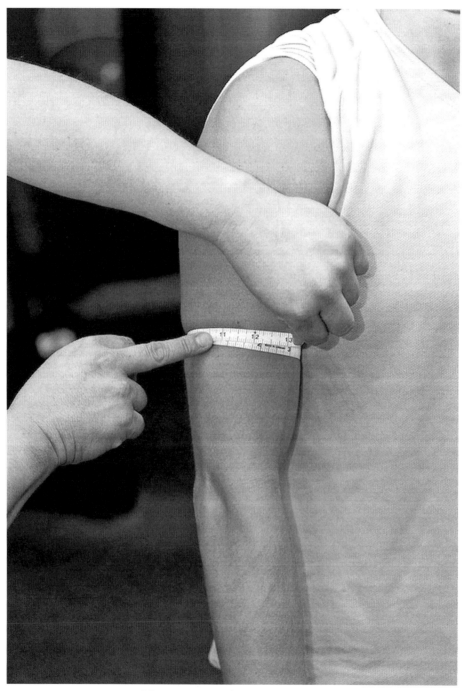
Upper arm girth measurement.

Performing Fitness Assessments and Reassessments

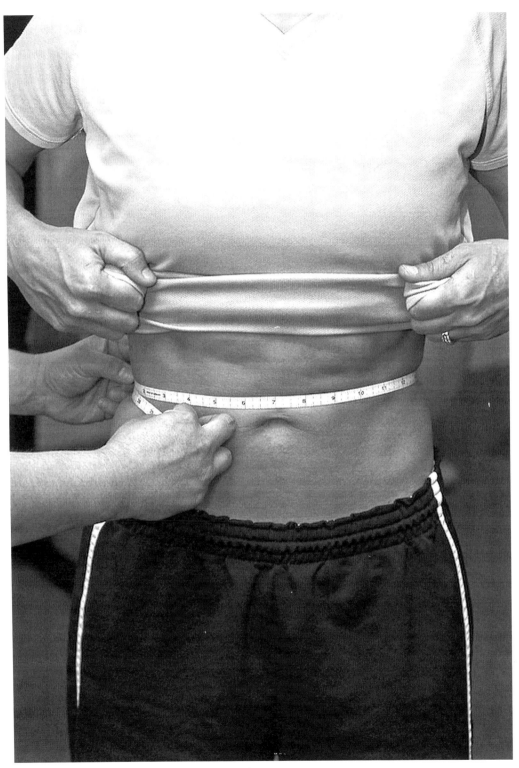

Waist girth measurement.

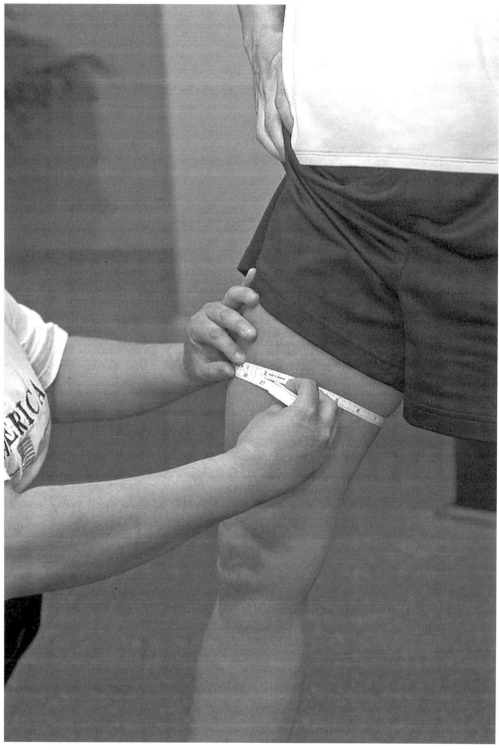

Thigh girth measurement.

Performing Fitness Assessments and Reassessments

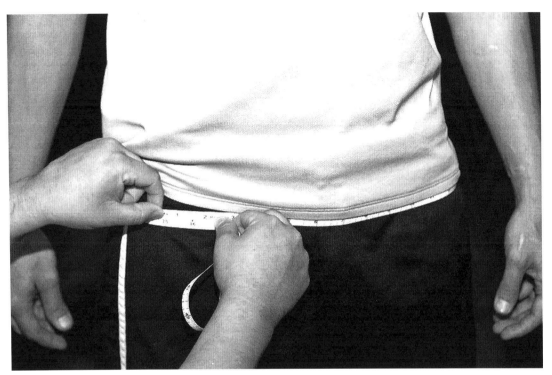

Hips girth measurement.

Girth Measurements

Girth Location	Girth Measurement (inches)
Chest (across the nipples; arms should be relaxed and down to the side)	
Abdominal (the point at which the belly is largest; generally, but not necessarily, at the level of the belly button)	
Waist (at the narrowest point of the waist/mid-section, or if that is unknown, at the midpoint between the last rib and the top of the hip bone, iliac crest)	
Hips (at widest area of buttocks and hips)	

Right thigh (midway between knee and hip)	
Left thigh (midway between knee and hip)	
Right upper arm (midway between elbow and acromium, the boney process on top of the shoulder)	
Left upper arm (midway between elbow and acromium)	
Left ankle (right above the end of the tibia/fibula bones)	
Right ankle (right above the end of the tibia/fibula bones)	
Neck (at the Adam's apple)	

Because of the relationship between abdominal obesity and elevated risk of chronic disease, waist circumference alone can be used to classify your health risk. Identify your risk, using the following table.

Waist Circumference in Inches and Centimeters (cm)		
Risk Category	Females	Males
Very low	< 28.5 (< 70 cm)	< 31.5 (< 80 cm)
Low	28.5-35.0 (70-89 cm)	31.5-39.0 (80-99 cm)
High	35.5-43.0 (90-109 cm)	39.5-47.0 (100-120 cm)
Very high	> 43.5 (110 cm)	> 47.0 (120 cm)

Source: Adapted from *ACSM's Guidelines for Exercise Testing and Prescription* [1].

Performing Fitness Assessments and Reassessments

LABORATORY WORK-UP

If you've never had a comprehensive laboratory work-up or it's been more than two years since you've had one, I highly recommend that you make an appointment with your primary care physician to get this accomplished. Often, we walk around with conditions we don't even know we have because there are no major side effects. High cholesterol, hypothyroidism, and abnormal blood glucose levels, which may suggest diabetes, are just a few examples of conditions that can be identified by appropriate laboratory tests.

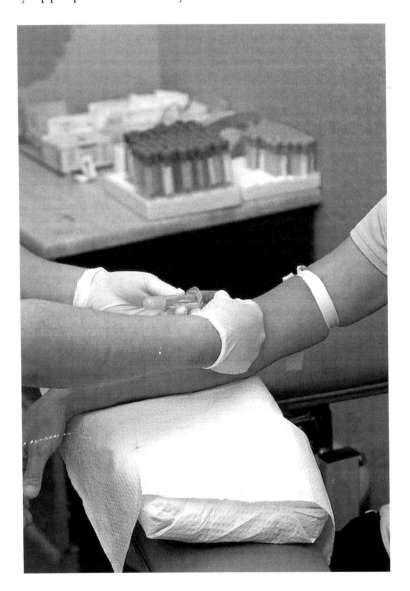

You should ask your physician for a comprehensive metabolic panel. This is a standard panel of 14 blood tests often ordered as part of a routine annual physical. You will need to fast for 10-12 hours prior to having a comprehensive metabolic lab panel done, meaning you should not consume any food or caloric beverages for 10-12 hours prior to getting your lab work-up. Medications are generally okay to take, provided you don't have to take them with food, but you should ask your physician if there is any medication you should temporarily stop.

LIPID PANEL

Included in a comprehensive metabolic panel is a full lipid panel. A lipid panel is a group of blood tests that measures lipids (fats) in your body. Lipids include total cholesterol and triglycerides. Triglycerides are a type of fat the body uses for energy. Cholesterol is used by the body to build cells and produce hormones. Not only will the panel measure your total cholesterol, but it will break it down into your high density lipoproteins (HDL), low density lipoproteins (LDL), very low density lipoproteins (VLDL), ratio of total cholesterol to HDL, and LDL to HDL ratio. Lipid disorders, particularly too much cholesterol, which can cause plaque build-up in the arteries, may lead to life-threatening illnesses such as stroke, heart attack, or heart disease. The desirable, acceptable, and undesirable ranges for cholesterol and triglycerides are listed in the following table.

Desirable, Acceptable, and Undesirable Ranges for Cholesterol and Triglycerides

Total cholesterol
   Desirable < 200 mg/dL
   Borderline high = 200-239 mg/dL
   High ≥ 240 mg/dL

HDL cholesterol
   High or desirable > 60 mg/dL
   Acceptable = 40-60 mg/dL
   Low or undesirable < 40 mg/dL

Total cholesterol-to-HDL ratio
   Desirable = 5:1 or less
   Undesirable = more than 5:1

LDL cholesterol
   Optimal < 100 mg/dL
   Near optimal = 100-129 mg/dL
   Borderline high = 130-159 mg/dL
   High = 160 - 189 mg/dL
   Very high ≥ 190 mg/dL

VLDL cholesterol
   Optimal < 130 mg/dL
   Borderline high = 130-159 mg/dL
   High ≥ 160 mg/dL

Triglycerides
   Optimal < 150 mg/dL
   Borderline high = 150-199 mg/dL
   High = 200-499 mg/dL
   Very high ≥ 500 mg/dL

Source: Values from the National Cholesterol Education Program (NCEP) of the National Institutes of Health (NIH) [5].

FASTING BLOOD GLUCOSE LEVEL

A fasting blood glucose level is often one of the first tests performed to check for diabetes. This test should be done first thing in the morning after not eating for 8-12 hours. This test can be done with a home monitoring device or in a physician's office. The American Diabetes Association's categorization of fasting blood glucose levels follows [6]:

- Optimal < 100 mg/dL
- Borderline high = 100-126 mg/dL
- High ≥ 126 mg/dL

A1C TEST

If you are diabetic or think you might have diabetes, an A1c test is the best method of determining disease status. This measures the amount of glycohemoglobin in the red blood cells. You don't have to fast for this test, and it doesn't matter what your blood glucose level is at the time of the test. The key advantage of this test is that it will identify your average blood glucose level over the past two to three months versus the level on a single day (i.e., the day of the test). Thus, if you haven't been monitoring your blood glucose levels appropriately, this test will reveal how well controlled your diabetes has been. The higher the A1c, the higher the risk of developing complications related to diabetes. The normal A1c range is 4-6 percent [7].

THYROID FUNCTION

It is also important to know if your thyroid is functioning properly. Normal thyroid levels range between 0.2 and 5.5 mU/L. Values greater than 5.5 mU/L signal low thyroid hormone and possible hypothyroidism. Hypothyroidism can cause weight gain because of an adverse effect on metabolism, causing it to be sluggish and low. This range is very broad; thus, some physicians believe the upper limit of the established "normal" range is too high. The thyroid stimulating hormone (TSH) test is often used to determine whether or not there is a deficiency in the thyroid gland hormone output. A TSH value of more than 2.03 mU/L may indicate lower-than-optimal thyroid hormone function [8]. Despite understanding what the normative values for your lab results are, it is always best to review the results with your primary care provider.

FLEXIBILITY ASSESSMENTS

Remember that flexibility is the ability to move a muscle or group of muscles surrounding a joint through the full range of motion. There are several different flexibility assessments you can perform. These can be accomplished by directly measuring a joint's range of motion or indirectly measuring a static distance in linear units. Several different flexibility assessments are described below. Select one or two to perform.

SIT-AND-REACH ASSESSMENT

Important: If you are unable to get down on the floor and back up again, do not perform this assessment.

AREA ASSESSED

This assessment measures hamstring and low-back flexibility.

REQUIRED EQUIPMENT

Acuflex I (modified sit-and-reach box) *or* a measuring tape is required. In addition, one other person is needed to help administer the test.

Performing Fitness Assessments and Reassessments

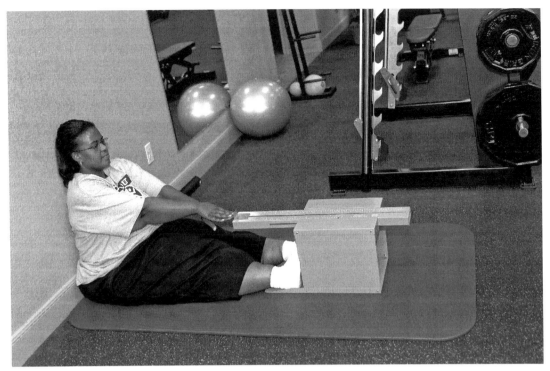

Starting position for sit and reach flexibility assessment.

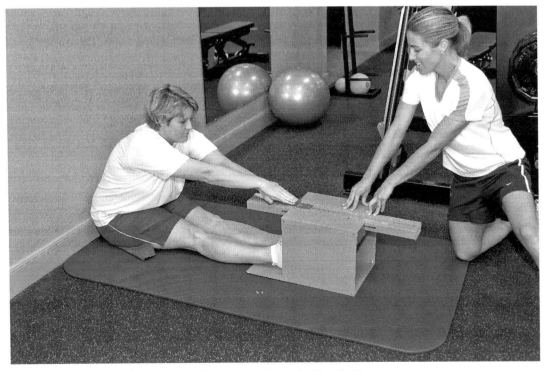

Final position for sit and reach flexibility assessment.

TESTING PROCEDURE

Be sure that the person being tested is properly warmed up prior to administering the test. After warming up, the individual takes his/her shoes off and sits down on the floor with his/her back flush against the wall and feet extended in front of the body. Then, he/she overlaps the hands so that the middle fingers are on top of one another and extends the hands out, keeping the back, hips, and shoulders against the wall and the legs fully extended. The person administering the test places the Acuflex box under the individual's feet, with the feet flat against the box. The metal L-shaped sliding mechanism should be placed at the end of the person's fingertips; this is the starting position. The testing administrator then holds the reach indicator firmly in place. If using a ruler or tape measure, the measuring device should be placed at the end of the person's fingers; this is zero (0) inches, or the starting position. The individual being tested is then allowed three attempts to reach forward (bringing the back and shoulders off the wall) as far as possible while keeping his/her legs flat against the floor (no bending of the knees). As the individual reaches forward, he/she holds the position at the end of the reach for 1-2 seconds. The testing administrator then determines the number of inches reached on each attempt, and the longest measurement is the individual's score. This sit-and-reach measurement determines one's degree of flexibility. The goal is to strive toward ranking in the 99th percentile.

Record your sit-and-reach score:_____ inches

ASSESSMENT SCORING RESULTS

Refer to the following table to determine your percentile ranking: _____
_____ percentile

Percentile Ranks for the Modified Sit-and-Reach Test: Men (Inches)

Percentile Rank	Age						
	10-14	15-19	20-29	30-39	40-49	50-59	60+
99	18.3	21.2	23.5	20.8	18.6	19.4	19.2
95	17.1	18.5	19.3	17.4	`6.8	16.4	17.0
90	16.4	17.5	17.9	16.3	15.5	15.5	15.5
80	15.7	16.3	17.3	14.9	14.5	13.5	14.5
70	14.8	15.5	16.2	13.9	13.5	12.5	13.8
60	13.3	14.5	15.3	13.3	12.9	11.6	12.5
50	12.2	13.6	14.3	12.3	12.3	10.6	12.3
40	11.0	12.6	13.8	11.5	11.4	10.0	11.7
30	10.3	11.8	13.0	10.5	10.8	9.3	10.3
20	9.1	10.8	11.8	8.4	10.0	8.5	9.3
10	8.3	9.0	10.3	7.0	8.0	7.4	8.8
5	7.4	8.5	9.3	6.7	7.3	5.4	7.5

Source: Adapted from The Assessment of Muscular Flexibility Test Protocols and National Flexibility Norms for the Modified Sit and Reach Test [9].

Percentile Ranks for the Modified Sit-and-Reach Test: Women (Inches)

Percentile Rank	Age						
	10-14	15-19	20-29	30-39	40-49	50-59	60+
99	22.7	23.0	23.7	22.1	22.0	19.4	18.2
95	21.2	20.6	20.8	17.9	17.5	16.6	15.6
90	18.7	18.8	19.7	17.0	16.9	15.9	15.5
80	17.6	17.8	18.3	16.8	16.0	13.9	14.3
70	17.0	16.7	17.0	16.1	15.0	13.5	13.0
60	16.5	15.8	16.2	15.0	14.2	12.5	10.5
50	15.8	15.3	15.5	14.3	13.0	11.5	9.8
40	14.8	14.8	14.8	13.6	12.5	10.3	9.5
30	13.8	13.8	14.0	12.5	12.0	9.8	9.2
20	13.0	12.8	13.0	11.1	10.7	8.5	7.7
10	11.8	11.6	11.9	9.0	8.6	7.5	5.9
5	10.6	10.3	10.7	8.0	8.0	6.0	3.0

Source: Adapted from The Assessment of Muscular Flexibility Test Protocols and National Flexibility Norms for the Modified Sit and Reach Test [9].

90-DEGREE FLEXIBILITY ASSESSMENT
AREA ASSESSED

This assessment measures hamstring and low back flexibility.

REQUIRED EQUIPMENT

The assessment requires use of a goniometer (a protractor could be used, if you don't have access to a goniometer) and a stiff table, bed, couch, or floor mat on the floor. In addition, one other person is needed to help administer the assessment. Two additional people would be ideal for this assessment (one to life the leg and the other to measure the angle on the goniometer), but it can be accomplished with one other person.

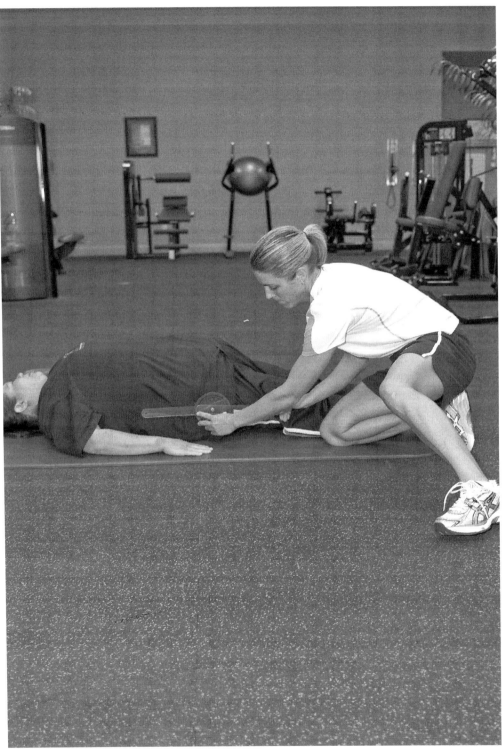

Starting position for 90-degree flexibility assessment.

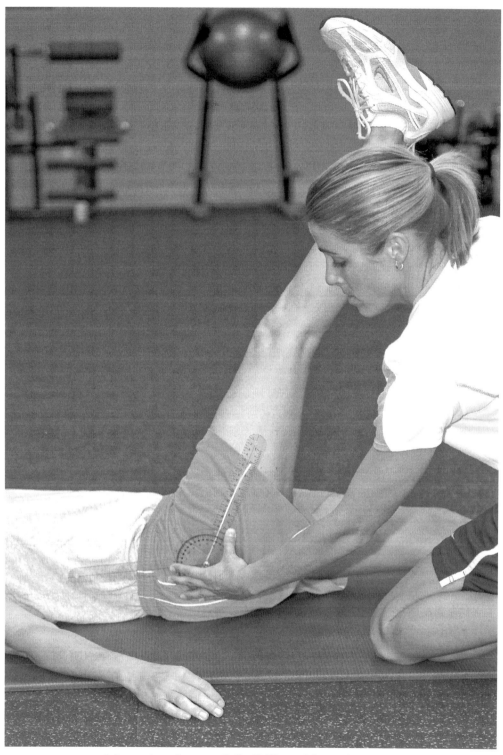

Measuring degree of flexibility with goniometer.

TESTING PROCEDURE

This assessment involves two trials in which the test administrator lifts one leg of the individual being tested. Be sure that the individual being tested is properly warmed up prior to the first trial. The individual starts in a supine (lying on back) position with both legs outstretched and the hands placed by the side, palms down. Both legs should be kept straight and the knee of the leg that remains on the table, bed, or mat while the other leg is lifted should not bend or leave the mat. Likewise, the leg being lifted by the test administrator should be kept straight, with no bend in the knee, while the administrator gradually pulls the leg up until the participant cannot stretch any further (being careful not to overstretch the muscle). Before the administrator pulls the leg up, he/she must palpate the individual's hip bone and place the middle (pivot joint) of the goniometer at the hip joint. If using a protractor, the administrator places the middle of the protractor at the hip joint; the bottom of the protractor should be parallel to the mat, floor, or bed. Once this has been accomplished, the administrator pulls up on the leg and measures the angle between the femur and the middle of the torso. The angle measured is then recorded. This assessment process is repeated for a second trial and the best result (smallest angle) is the individual's score.

90-degree flexibility score:_____ degrees

ASSESSMENT SCORING RESULTS

This is a pass/fail assessment. If the individual's measurement (angle measured between the femur and middle of the torso) is less than 90 degrees, he/she passes. A score of more than 90 degrees is failing. Thus, the goal is to have a score less than 90 degrees. If you're not there yet, you simply need to start stretching on a daily basis. Remember, if you have good flexibility, you will be able to do your daily activities with ease and prevent injuries while exercising. It is never too late to start stretching.

SHOULDER FLEXIBILITY ASSESSMENT I
AREA ASSESSED

This assessment determines an individual's degree of shoulder flexibility.

Rx Fitness for Weight Loss: The Medically Sound Solution to Get Fit and Save Your Life

REQUIRED EQUIPMENT

The assessment requires use of a stick, towel, or rope and a measuring tape. One additional person is needed to help administer the test.

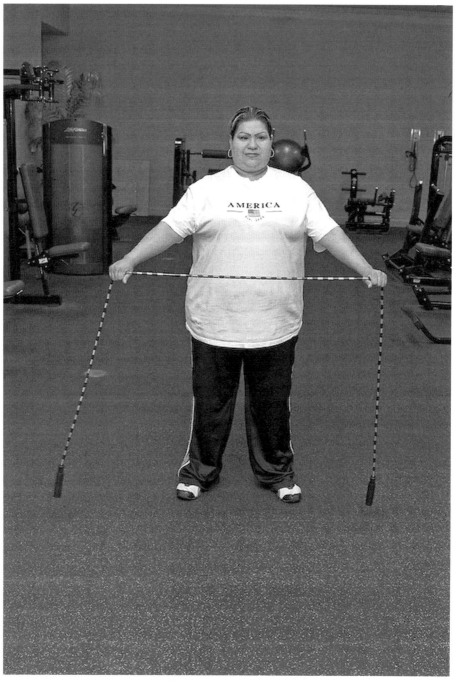

Shoulder flexibility assessment I starting position.

Performing Fitness Assessments and Reassessments

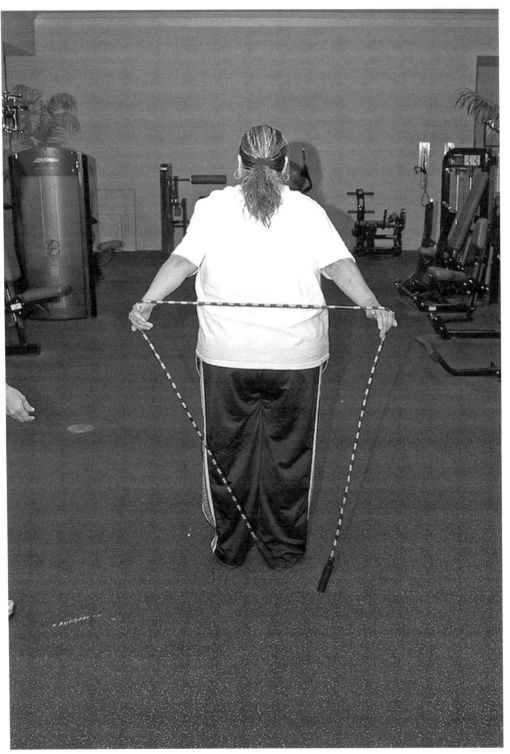

Shoulder flexibility assessment I with rope and arms behind the back.

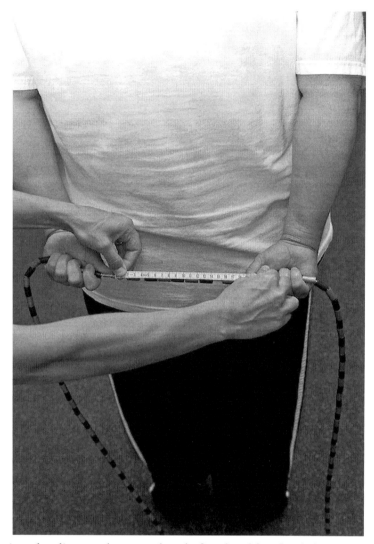
Measuring the distance between hands for shoulder flexibility assessment I.

TESTING PROCEDURES

The individual being assessed starts by holding the rope, towel, or stick with both hands out in front of the body. The hands should be wide apart, with the palms pronated, or facing downward. Then he/she lifts the rope, towel, or stick, over the head and behind the back while maintaining the grip on the object. The object should be against the back. Next, the person inches the hands until they cannot be moved any closer. Then, the test administrator measures the distance between the hands to the closest 1/4 inch. This measurement is the test score.

Shoulder flexibility score:_____ inches between hands

ASSESSMENT SCORING RESULTS

There is no normative data for this shoulder flexibility test. The score is simply recorded and reassessments should be accomplished every three to four months. If the distance measured in reassessments becomes smaller, shoulder flexibility has increased (improved).

SHOULDER FLEXIBILITY ASSESSMENT II
AREA ASSESSED

This assessment determines an individual's degree of shoulder flexibility.

REQUIRED EQUIPMENT

A measuring tape and one person to administer the test are required.

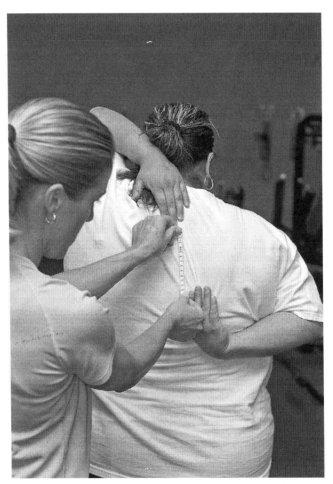

Measuring the distance between fingers for shoulder flexibility assessment II.

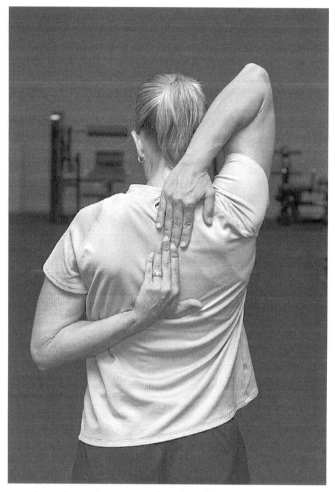

Fingers touch and passing score for shoulder flexibility assessment II.

TESTING PROCEDURES

Put one arm over your head and reach down your back. Put your opposite arm behind your back and reach up toward the other hand. Then the testing administrator measures the smallest distance between the fingers of each opposing hand. This measurement is your score.

Shoulder flexibility II score:_____ inches between two fingers

ASSESSMENT SCORING RESULTS

This is a pass/fail test. If you are able to touch your fingers on each hand or one hand with the other hand, you pass. If you cannot do this, you fail and simply need to stretch more frequently, especially the shoulders, and then reassess in three to four months. The closer the hands get together or the shorter the distance between the two hands, the better your shoulder flexibility.

CARDIOVASCULAR ASSESSMENTS

A cardiovascular fitness assessment helps identify your current cardiovascular fitness level—that is, your "heart health." There are several different types of cardiovascular fitness tests. Some of these tests must be administered by a qualified fitness staff and/or physician, while others can be performed in the comfort of your own home. Only three different types of assessments are described below, but understand that there are several more to choose from.

VO2 MAX CARDIOVASCULAR ASSESSMENT

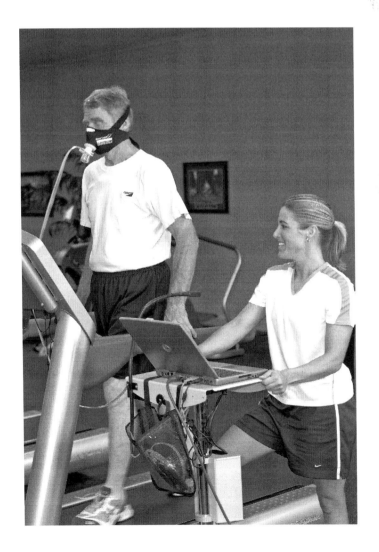

One type of maximal cardiovascular fitness (cardio/aerobic) assessment is called the VO2 max test. This is a form of metabolic testing and must be administered by a fitness professional. Also referred to as *indirect calorimetry*, it is one of the most accurate cardiovascular fitness assessments because it is individual to each person. Due to its individuality, it takes the guesswork out of evaluating and prescribing cardio/aerobic exercise. So what is VO2 max and what does it mean? *VO2 max* is defined as the maximal volume of oxygen uptake measured in mL/kg/min. When you exercise aerobically, you must utilize oxygen in order to burn calories. The more efficient your body is at utilizing the oxygen you take in, the higher the level of your cardiovascular fitness—in other words, the healthier your heart. You see, if you can effectively utilize the oxygen you breathe in, your heart doesn't have to work as hard to get the oxygen to the cells in your body. All the cells, muscles, and organs in your body need oxygen in order to metabolize or burn calories.

Keep in mind that your body burns primarily fat or carbohydrate for fuel in both a resting and active state. In light of this fact, you might be wondering why so many people have such a hard time burning fat. Chances are that they are taking in more calories than their bodies are burning and they haven't trained their bodies to be efficient at burning fat. Your fitness level determines how effectively your body uses fat as a fuel source during exercise. Generally speaking, your body is better at utilizing fat at low to moderate exercise intensities. The reason for this is because one needs more oxygen to metabolize fat, and for most of us, this can be accomplished better at lower intensities. However, the more fit you become, the better your body can metabolize fat at higher exercise intensities. This is part of the reason why fit people tend to stay leaner; their bodies are simply better at burning fat. The other thing that happens when one is more fit is that the body burns more fat at higher intensities and for longer durations. Some VO2 max assessments reveal how many total calories and what percentage of those calories are fat at every minute during the test in relationship to your heart rate. With this type of information, you can easily set up an exercise program that maximizes your body's ability to burn fat during exercise. See Chapter 7 for details on how to set up your exercise program to maximize fat loss.

Your anaerobic threshold can also be determined by VO2 max testing. The anaerobic threshold is the point at which your body is no longer utilizing oxygen to burn calories—thus *anaerobic*, meaning without oxygen. At this point you are burning straight carbohydrates because your body must use oxygen to metabolize fat. As I mentioned previously, a fitness professional needs to administer this assessment. Call your local fitness centers or health and wellness clinics to see if anyone in your area performs this type of testing.

I have personally administered thousands of metabolic tests over the past four years, and I highly recommend that every able person undergo this testing, specifically the VO2 max test. If you want to take your fitness to the next level and are serious about your weight loss, this test is definitely for you. There are several health and fitness facilities that perform metabolic testing. Just make sure your testing administer is educated, qualified, and experience in the field of exercise.

SUBMAXIMAL VO2 ASSESSMENTS

Submaximal VO2 testing is another method of assessing cardiovascular fitness. This test uses heart rate performance to estimate the body's ability to utilize oxygen. There are many different submaximal tests. Three field tests that you should be able to accomplish in the comfort of your own home or a local park are subsequently described. If you're taking a beta blocker or any other medication that significantly lowers your blood pressure, do not perform the Rockport 1-Mile Walking Test, since medications that significantly lower your heart rate will throw off the VO2 score simply because the heart rate is calculated into the VO2 equation. If you are taking a beta blocker, perform either the 1-mile walk for time, or if you're in better shape, the 1½ mile run test.

ROCKPORT 1-MILE FITNESS WALKING TEST

For this test, you need to mark off a relatively flat route that is 1 mile in distance [1]. A 1-mile route in a park or local track is ideal, but you can also perform this test on a treadmill. In addition to your 1-mile route, you will need a heart rate monitor. Be sure to warm up before performing this test. Once you've properly warmed up, you will be walking 1 mile as fast as possible. Your heart rate will be taken during the final minute of the assessment or for the first 10 seconds immediately following the completion of the walk. It is very important to record the time in minutes it took to walk 1 mile as well as the average heart rate during the last minute of the walk. Your VO2 max is then estimated using the equation below. This equation uses your gender, age, weight, walk time, and heart rate as factors in estimating your cardiovascular fitness.

Record time in minutes to walk 1 mile: _____ minutes

Record average heart rate for last minute of walk: _____ bpm

Equation to estimate VO2 max using the 1-mile walking test [10]:

VO2 max (mL/kg/min) = 132.853 − 0.1692 (body mass in kg) − 1.3877 (age in years) + 6.315 (gender) − 3.2649 (time in minutes) − 0.1565 (heart rate)

Note: 2.2 kg = 1 lb; gender = 1 for males, 0 for females

Now that you know your cardiovascular fitness score, you're probably wondering if this is poor, good, or excellent. Refer to the following table to determine your overall heart health [11].

VO2 Max Values for Men and Women

Male

Age	Very Poor	Poor	Fair	Good	Excellent	Superior
13-19	0-34.9	35.0-38.3	38.4-45.1	45.2-50.9	51.0-55.9	56.0+
20-29	0-32.9	33.0-36.4	36.5-42.4	42.5-46.4	46.5-52.4	52.5+
30-39	0-31.4	31.5-35.4	35.5-40.9	41.0-44.9	45.0-49.4	49.5+
40-49	0-30.2	30.2-33.5	33.6-38.9	39.0-43.7	43.8-48.0	48.1+
50-59	0-26.0	26.1-30.9	31.0-35.7	35.8-40.9	41.0-45.3	45.4+
60+	0-20.4	20.5-26.0	26.1-32.2	32.3-36.4	36.5-44.2	44.3+

Female

Age	Very Poor	Poor	Fair	Good	Excellent	Superior
13-19	0-24.9	25.0-30.9	31.0-34.9	35.0-38.9	39.0-41.9	42.0+
20-29	0-23.5	23.6-28.9	29.0-32.9	33.0-36.9	37.0-41.0	41.1+
30-39	0-22.7	22.8-26.9	27.0-31.4	31.5-35.6	35.7-40.0	40.1+
40-49	0-20.9	21.0-24.4	24.5-28.9	29.0-32.8	32.9-36.9	37.0+
50-59	0-20.1	20.2-22.7	22.8-26.9	27.0-31.4	31.5-35.7	35.8+
60+	0-17.4	17.5-20.1	20.2-24.4	24.5-30.2	30.3-31.4	31.5+

Source: From *The Aerobics Way* [11].

If you are taking a beta blocker or any other medication that affects the heart rate, or if you do not have access to a heart rate monitor, use the time in minutes in the following table to determine your cardiovascular fitness.

Cardiorespiratory Fitness Rating Based on Time in Minutes for 1-Mile Walking Test

Rating	Men under 40	Men over 40	Women under 40	Women over 40
Excellent	13:00 or less	14:00 or less	13:30 or less	14:30 or less
Good	13:0-15:30	14:01-16:30	13:31-16:00	14:31-17:00
Average	15:31-18:00	16:31-19:00	16:01-18:00	17:01-19:30
Below average	18:01-19:30	19:01-21:30	18:31-20:00	19:31-22:00
Low	19:31 or more	21:31 or more	20:01 or more	22:01 or more

Source: From *The Cooper Institute Physical Fitness Specialist Course and Certification Manual* [12].

MODIFIED CARDIOVASCULAR FITNESS ASSESSMENT

If you don't feel you can walk a full mile or you simply cannot walk due to physical limitations, choose a piece of cardio exercise equipment that you can use within your limitations. Designate a set work rate and time in minutes and wear a heart rate monitor during the test. After you've properly warmed up, begin the test by exercising for the allotted time period and work rate. The goal is to cover as much distance as possible in the allotted time. Record this distance along with the work load or intensity (e.g., level 5 on the recumbent bike) you had the equipment set at. Also record your average heart rate for the duration of the test. Retest using the same exact protocol in two to three months; if you were able to cover more distance and/or your average heart rate has decreased, you have definitely improved your cardiovascular fitness level.

1.5-MILE RUN TEST

If you are relatively fit and jog or run for your cardio exercise, this test may be more suitable for you. This test is not recommended for unfit individuals or beginners. Be sure you are able to run and cover a distance of 1.5 miles. If you are not able to do both of these things, perform the 1-mile walking test or modified cardiovascular fitness assessment previously described. The objective of this test is to cover a distance of 1.5 miles in the shortest amount of time. Be sure to properly warm up prior to the test. Although the protocols of this test do not specify whether or not you can use a treadmill, I suggest using one, since this is the easiest method to accurately determine how far you've gone and how much time it took you to cover the 1.5-mile distance. If you are not using a treadmill, you need to identify or designate a route that is clearly marked off at 1.5 miles. A 400-meter track would be ideal: four laps equal mile; therefore, six laps need to be run to complete this test. Refer to the following table to determine your fitness rating.

1.5-Mile Run Fitness Rating for Women (Time in Minutes)

Category	Age 20-29	Age 30-39	Age 40-49	Age 50-59	Age 60-69	Age 70-79
Superior	9:23-10:20	9:52-11:08	10:09-11:35	11:34-13:16	12:25-14:28	12:25-14:33
Excellent	10:59-11:56	11:43-12:53	12:25-13:38	13:58-15:14	15:32-16:46	16:06-18:05
Good	12:07-13:25	13:08-14:33	13:58-15:17	15:47-17:19	17:34-18:52	18:39-20:54
Fair	13:58-15:05	14:33-15:56	15:56-17:11	17:38-19:10	19:29-20:55	21:45-23:47
Poor	15:32-17:11	16:43-18:18	17:38-19:43	19:43-21:57	22:03-23:55	24:54-27:17
Very poor	17:53-25:17	19:01-25:10	20:49-27:55	22:53-30:34	25:02-33:05	27:55-37:26

Source: Adapted from *The Cooper Institute Physical Fitness Specialist Course and Certification Manual* [12].

1.5-Mile Run Fitness Rating for Men (Time in Minutes)

Category	Age 20-29	Age 30-39	Age 40-49	Age 50-59	Age 60-69	Age 70-79
Superior	8:22-9:10	8:49-9:31	9:02-9:47	9:31-10:27	10:09-11:20	10:27-12:25
Excellent	9:34-10:08	9:52-10:38	10:09-11:09	11:09-12:08	12:10-13:25	13:25-14:52
Good	10:34-11:27	10:59-11:49	11:32-12:25	12:37-13:53	13:58-15:20	15:38-17:37
Fair	11:34-12:29	11:58-12:53	12:53-13:50	13:58-15:14	15:53-17:19	18:05-19:43
Poor	12:53-13:58	13:25-14:33	14:10-15:32	15:53-17:30	17:49-20:13	20:28-23:55
Very poor	14:33-20:55	15:14-20:55	16:09-22:22	18:22-27:08	21:34-31:59	25:49-33:30

Source: Adapted from *The Cooper Institute Physical Fitness Specialist Course and Certification Manual* [12].

Record all of your cardiovascular fitness score results in the following chart. Stay consistent with your exercise program and reassess your fitness level every three to four months.

Record of Fitness Level

Type of Assessment	Assessment Date	Score (mL/kg/min or Minutes)	Score Category (Superior, Excellent, Good, Average, Below Average, Low)	Notes
VO2 max				
Rockport 1-mile walk				
1-mile walk for time				
Modified cardiovascular fitness assessment (record equipment, time, level, and distance covered)				
1.5-mile run for time				

MUSCULAR STRENGTH ASSESSMENTS

There are four simple muscular strength assessments you can perform in the comfort of your own home: a wall sit, timed chair squats, 1-minute push-ups, and 1-minute knee taps or sit-ups. These assessments target one's lower body strength, upper body strength, and abdominal strength consecutively.

LOWER BODY STRENGTH ASSESSMENTS

WALL SIT

This tests your lower body strength. Do not perform this assessment if you have any type of knee condition or limitation, since it simulates a squat and may cause further knee pain or discomfort.

You need a stop watch and a wall to perform this test. Start with your back against the wall, your feet about shoulder width apart, and the heels of your feet positioned approximately 2 feet out away from the wall. Squat down until your thighs are parallel to the floor. This is your starting position (see the following photograph).

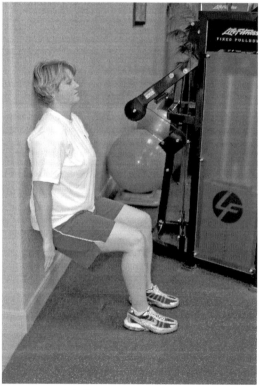

Wall squat assessment.

Now that you are in your wall-sit starting position, start the stop watch. You need to keep your back pressed against the wall, and your arms must be down at your side. In other words, you can't lean on your legs with your hands. The goal is to stay in this wall-sit position for as long as possible. Turn the stop watch off when you can no longer hold yourself up and/or your buttocks touch the floor. If you reach 5 minutes with good form, you've maxed out this assessment.

Wall sit score:_____minutes

1-MINUTE CHAIR SQUATS

This also tests your lower body strength. Do not perform this assessment if you have any type of knee condition or limitation, since this assessment may cause further knee pain or discomfort.

You need a stop watch and a chair to perform this test. Start by standing in front of the chair, with your heels positioned about 2 inches in front of the seat of the chair. You should stand in neutral alignment (feet shoulder width apart, shoulders back, chest out, head up, and chin parallel to the floor). See the photograph on the following page for your starting position. You perform the assessment by squatting back into the chair. As you lower yourself toward the chair, be sure to bend at the waist, sticking your buttocks out and then bending the knees. Also, your back should remain flat or straight; do not round your back as you perform this exercise. The key is to sit back "into" the exercise: Imagine using a public toilet and having to squat or hover over the toilet seat without touching it. I often refer to this test movement as the *public toilet squat*. Now, for this assessment, you need to barely touch the seat of the chair. Do not release all of your weight into the chair. Each time you touch the seat of the chair is one repetition. The goal is to perform as many repetitions as possible in 1 minute.

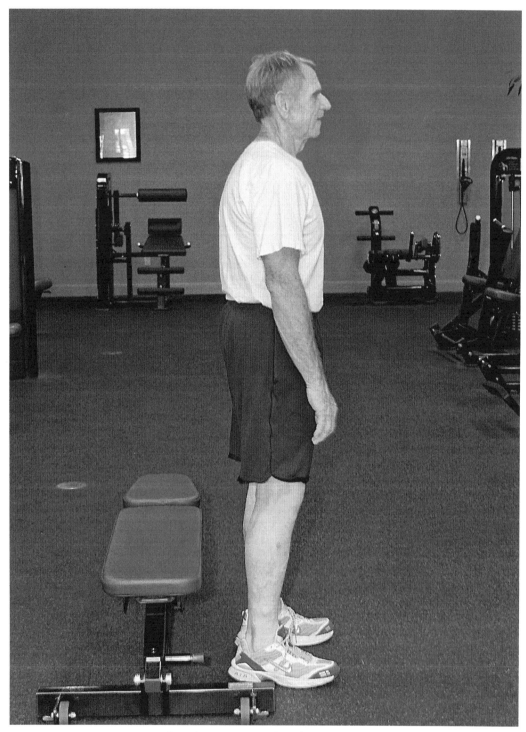
Starting position for chair squat.

Performing Fitness Assessments and Reassessments

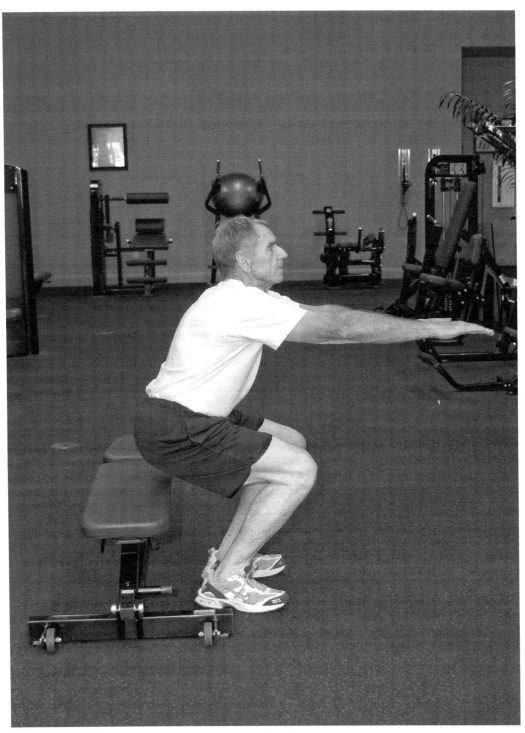

Final position for chair squat.

Now that you understand the starting position and how to perform the chair squat, begin the assessment. Position yourself in the starting position. Start the stopwatch. Then, perform as many chair squats as you can in 1 minute. Remember, if you don't touch the seat, it doesn't count. The assessment is over after 1 minute elapses. Record your score below.

Chair squats:_____repetitions

Reassess either one of these lower body strength assessments every three to four months. If you are able to hold yourself up for a longer period of time during the wall squat or are able to perform more repetitions in 1 minute during the chair squat, your lower body strength is improving.

UPPER BODY STRENGTH ASSESSMENT

1-MINUTE PUSHUPS

This will test your upper body muscular strength. Do not perform this assessment if you have any type of shoulder condition or limitation, since it simulates a chest press and may cause further shoulder discomfort or pain.

You'll need a stopwatch and a yoga block (or fluffy pillow) for this assessment. You can perform this one of two ways: either the full pushup version or the modified version. The starting and finishing positions are shown in the following photographs. Whichever version you choose, be sure your back is straight and your chest lowers to the yoga block or pillow for each repetition. Place the pillow or yoga block directly under your chest. You can only rest in the up position, arms extended with the back straight. Each time your chest lowers down and touches the pillow or yoga block is one repetition. The goal is to perform as many repetitions as possible in 1 minute.

Performing Fitness Assessments and Reassessments

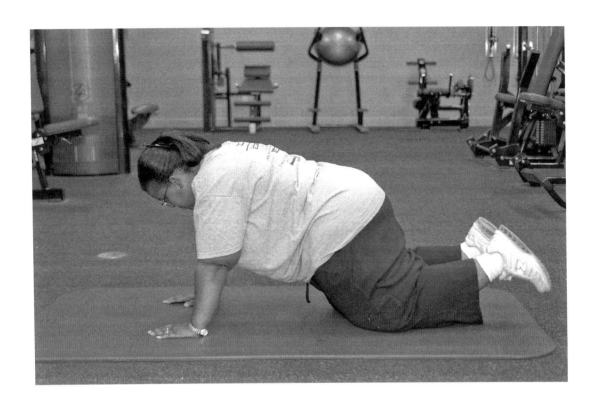

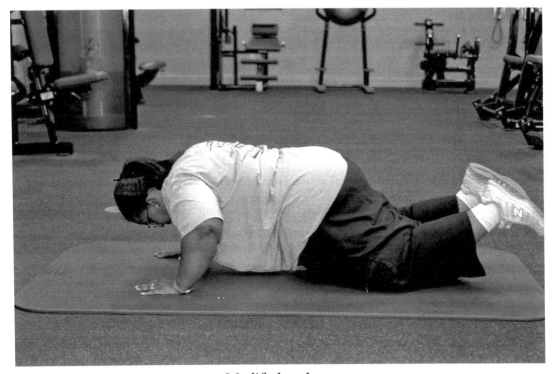

Modified pushups.

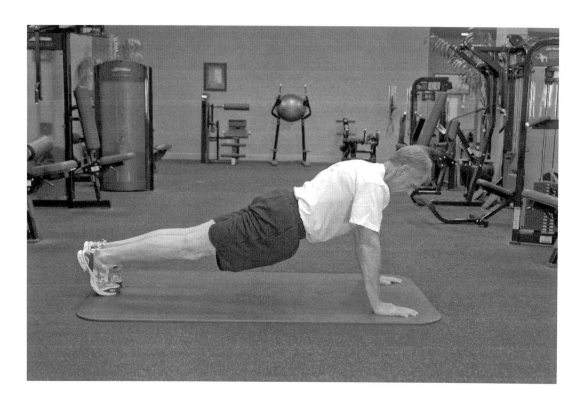

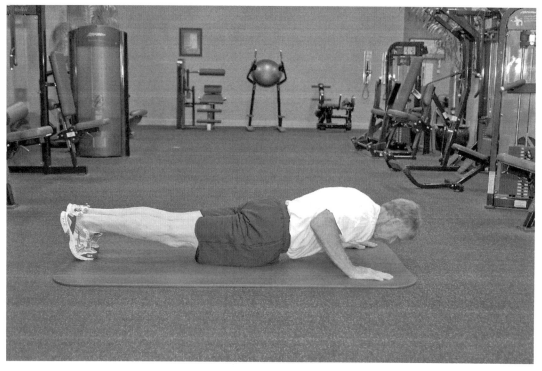

Full pushups.

1-minute pushup score:_____ repetitions

Reassess every three to four months. If you are able to increase the total number of pushups performed in 1 minute, your upper body muscular strength and endurance have increased.

ABDOMINAL STRENGTH ASSESSMENT

1-MINUTE KNEE TAPS OR SIT-UPS

This will test your abdominal strength. Do not perform this assessment if you have any type of abdominal condition or limitation, such as a hernia, since it may cause further abdominal discomfort or pain.

You need a stopwatch for this assessment. The starting and finishing positions are shown in the following photographs. You can perform this assessment on the floor, your bed, or a stretch table. For the knee taps you'll need to keep your arms outstretched in front of your body throughout the assessment. Slowly crunch up and tap your knees with your fingertips each time you rise up. Every time you tap your knees is 1 repetition. Sit-ups begin with the arms folded across your chest. You can either place your feet under a secure object (e.g., couch) or have another person hold your feet. Slowly come up until the elbows touch the thighs. If you have to rest, you'll need to rest in the up position for sit-ups. The goal is to perform as many repetitions as possible in 1 minute.

1-minute knee tap score:_____ repetitions

1-minute sit-up score:_____ repetitions

Reassess every three to four months. If you are able to increase the total number of knee taps or sit-ups performed in one minute, you have increased your abdominal strength. If you are unable to do a full sit-up start with knee taps and then progress to sit-ups.

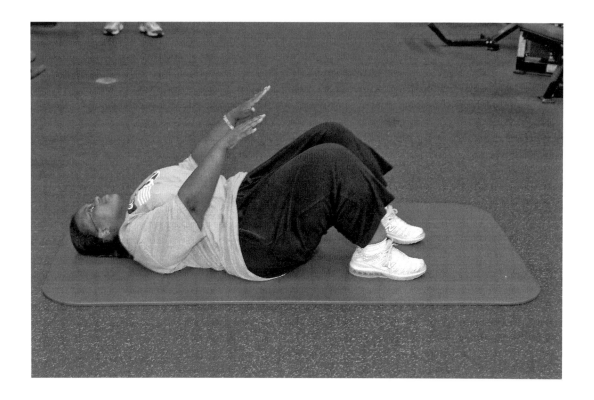

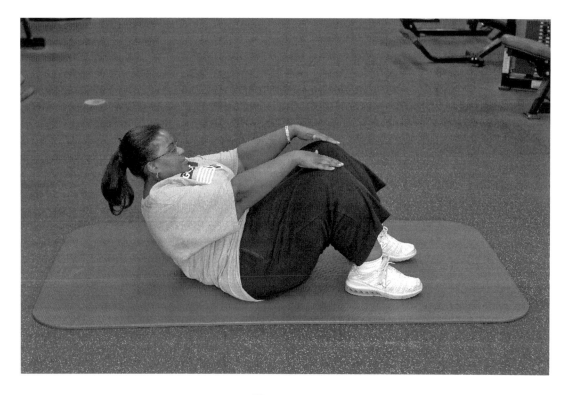

Knee taps.

REFERENCES

1. *ACSM's Guidelines for Exercise Testing and Prescription*, 7th Ed. Indianapolis: American College of Sports Medicine, 2006. Pp 44, 58, 61, 66-67, 69,70, 189-191, 298.
2. Boyle, Richard. Maintaining balance with age, 2002. Available at: www.ec-online.net/Knowledge/Article/balance.html; accessed July 17, 2007.
3. *Clinical Guidelines on the Identification, Evaluation, and Treatment of Overweight and Obesity in Adults. The Evidence Report: September* (Appendix V). Washington, DC: National Institutes of Health, 1987.
4. *Tanita Monitoring Your Health BF-679/BF-680W Body Fat Monitor Instruction Manual: 5.* Arlington, IL: Tanita Corporation, 2005.
5. National Institute of Health: National Cholesterol Education Program, 2007. Available at: www.webmd.com/cholesterol-management/Cholesterol-and-Triglycerides-Tests?page=3; accessed July 24, 2007.
6. *Diabetes A to Z: What You Need to Know About Diabetes—Simply Put*, 5th Ed. Alexandria, VA: American Diabetes Association, 2003. Pp 142, 143.
7. WebMD Medical Reference, 2005. Hemoglobin A1C test for diabetes. Available at: http://diabetes.webmd.com/guide/glycated-hemoglobin-test-hba1c; accessed July 24, 2007.
8. Life Extensions, 2006. Health concerns: thyroid regulation. Available at: www.lef.org/protocols/metabolic_health/thyroid_regulation_0.1.htm; accessed July 24, 2007.
9. Hoeger, Werner WK, and Hopkins, David R. The Assessment of Muscular Flexibility Test Protocols and National Flexibility Norms for the Modified Sit and Reach Test. In: Acuflex I (sit- and-reach box) user's manual, 2002.
10. Kline, GM, Porcari, JP, Hintermeister, R, et al. Estimation of VO2 max from a one-mile track walk, gender, age, and body weight. *Medicine and Science in Sports and Exercise* 1987;19(3):253-359.
11. Cooper, Kenneth. *The Aerobics Way* (VO2 max tables.) Dallas: Bantam Books, 1982.
12. Oddan, William E. Physical fitness assessments. In: *The Cooper Institute Physical Fitness Specialist Course and Certification Manual.* Dallas: The Cooper Institute, 2004. Pp 5, 13, 30-32.

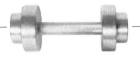

Part III

GOING THE "EXTRA MILE" TO GET RESULTS

Chapter 9
Doctors' Keys to Successful Weight Loss

A BARIATRICIAN'S PERSPECTIVE

This section identifies what it takes from a bariatrician's perspective to be successful in one's attempt to lose weight. The content of this chapter was extrapolated from an interview the author conducted with Dr. Tamyra Rogers on March 13, 2008. Dr. Rogers is a licensed physician who specializes in the causes, treatment, and prevention of obesity. She is board certified by the American Board of Bariatrics Medicine and Internal Medicine. Dr. Rogers owns and manages Dr. Rogers Wellness & Weight Loss Center in San Antonio, Texas. Previous to running her own clinic, she was the medical director for a multidisciplinary medical and surgical weight-loss program. She also directed the Northeast Methodist Metabolic Clinic as well as the Metabolic Clinic for the Tuba City Indian Medical Center. She's been practicing medicine for 11 years and has helped thousands of patients regain their health as well as their quality of life.

Over the years of practicing bariatric medicine (the medicine of weight loss), Dr. Rogers has witnessed amazing weight-loss achievements as well as some outright weight-loss failures among her patients. The reason for the pronounced disparity is that one's success depends largely on the individual. Dr. Rogers states that she, as a physician, can definitely help people lose weight, but the success of the endeavor rests primarily on the individual's own motivation and drive. People who come in with specific goals they are trying to achieve and who have a definite timeline for achieving their goals tend to be more successful.

Dr. Rogers has identified specific traits, characteristics, and tactics directly related to the success of individuals on a journey of weight loss. These keys to success are described in the following sections of this chapter.

REALIZE YOUR HABITS

Some people are more successful than others because they realize or understand how their habits have affected their weight gain or loss. "I really put people that are trying to lose weight into two distinct classifications," Rogers says. I see people who are morbidly obese as well as people who are moderately overweight. These two groups of people tend to view their habits a bit differently. People who are moderately overweight tend to be more successful, especially with medical weight loss. The reason for this is because they have less weight to lose, and more than likely, they gained weight due to an event in their life, e.g., a death in the family, birth of a child, entering college, working in a stressful environment, or recent move to a new house. Whatever the situation, moderately overweight people tend to recognize that they've gained the excess weight due to poor choices or habits they've developed over the course of whatever situation they are dealing with. Many of these people had relatively healthy habits before a particular event happened, but they allowed the situation to deter them from their regular routine. Once they recognize what they are doing, they can more easily change back to the healthy habits they had before the event occurred. Morbidly obese people, on the other hand, tend to have a much more difficult time changing the habits that have contributed to their weight gain. They have a difficult time believing in weight loss because they've failed at several different diets or weight-loss programs in the past and may have even gained more weight than they lost after getting off a diet. After numerous attempts, they usually easily fall back into their old, not-so-healthy habits and may even develop more unhealthy habits due to low self-esteem and self-confidence. This low emotional state can be exacerbated even more by each unsuccessful attempt to lose weight. For the morbidly obese, weight-loss surgery is often the best option because it rids them of the feeling of hunger that directly contributes to poor eating habits. This isn't to say that morbidly obese people can't be successful in weight loss, but these individuals must realize what their bad habits are and change these habits to foster weight loss. New, healthy habits must be established and be maintained for the rest of their lives. If you can confront your unhealthy habits and understand how you developed them, you'll have a better chance of weight-loss success.

Rogers claims that a patient's success is even better assured if the individual comes to her well-prepared—that is, the individual has filled out the clinic's questionnaire and has really thought hard about and understands what she or he is embarking on and the cause-effect factors in having become overweight. If the patient is an active participant in the initial medical consultation, the individual has a good chance of losing weight. Conversely, if the patient continually makes excuses for why he or she can't do the necessary things to lose weight, chances are that such a patient is not really ready to lose weight and any weight-loss endeavors are going to be very challenging.

CHANGE YOUR HABITS BUT DO SO INCREMENTALLY

We all have habits, some good, some not so good, and some just plain bad. The question is how can someone break unhealthy (bad) habits that contribute to weight gain? Dr. Rogers states that once you've identified the habits you need to change, it is best to gradually whittle them down instead of trying to cut them out suddenly. In other words, don't try to stop them "cold turkey" or suddenly drastically change what you've been doing for years. Incrementally change your unhealthy habits one step at a time. For example, if you eat out for all of your meals, chances are that you're not going to suddenly stop eating out. A more realistic approach would be to eat one of your meals at home or to bring your lunch to work versus always eating out for lunch. After you've been successful with your initial step for a month or two, then take another step and eat out only for dinner two or three times a week versus every night. Whatever the change may be, the key is to start slowly and incrementally transform your habits.

BELIEVE IN WEIGHT LOSS

The mental/psychological state of a patient plays a big role in the individual's success. Rogers states that patients must mentally "buy into" the methods and goals of a weight-loss program. There are so many different ways to lose weight out there—so many gimmicks. If the patient hasn't bought into a weight-loss program, she or he will easily deviate. Most people who commit themselves to a weight-loss plan will lose weight: It doesn't necessarily matter what the particular plan is; the level of commitment the individual has to the weight-loss program is the real key to success.

If you feel like you've tried every weight-loss program and never had success, Dr. Rogers would tell you that you've never really followed those programs. Rogers tends to dismiss someone's telling her they can't lose weight even when they're on a program. The only exception is someone who has an eating disorder. In this case, the patient has "messed up" their metabolism so severely that these programs tend not to work for them. However, for the majority of people, if they eat less, they will lose weight. If you take in fewer calories than your body burns in one day, you will lose weight. Rogers doesn't claim that these programs will allow you to maintain the weight you've lost once you stop a diet. You can't be on a diet forever, and most weight-loss diets don't teach you how to maintain your weight once you lose it. Your transition phase is extremely important in long-term maintenance of weight loss. One of the most important things with regard to transitioning from a diet is to be on a regular exercise program. Exercise is an absolute for the person that desires to keep the weight off long term. Not transitioning properly is why so many people tend to gain back a lot of the weight they lose from dieting.

The bottom line is that you have to mentally and physically "buy into" whatever weight-loss program you are on. If you are pessimistic or have doubts about the program, you will be a victim of "letdown." Believe in what you are doing and go for it!

GENETIC MAKEUP AFFECTS YOUR SUCCESS BUT DOES NOT RULE YOUR SUCCESS

Dr. Rogers definitely thinks people are genetically predisposed to become overweight or obese. Studies show that if your parents are obese, you have a much higher percentage of being obese because of the genetic makeup you inherited from them. The important thing to remember is that you "pull the trigger." You personally make the decision to eat what you are going to eat and whether you are going to exercise or not, and these decisions will make the real difference in your ability to combat the obesity gene. So, if you're predisposed to being obese, create an environment that fosters healthy habits. Do not create an obesity-promoting environment. Rogers says that if you do, you'll either become obese or place yourself in the extreme opposite position, possibly to the point of becoming anorexic or bulimic because you're so scared of becoming obese.

One important point Dr. Rogers makes is that someone who is obese and is genetically predisposed to obesity has a much greater rate of success with weight-loss surgery.

UNDERSTAND THAT EXERCISE AND DIET ARE KEYS TO LONG-TERM SUCCESS

Regular exercise and moderate intake of calories are crucial for long-term weight loss. Five hours a week of exercise is needed in order to maintain a healthy weight, and it is important to "change up" your exercise routine and align it with where you're at in your weight-loss goals. You should change up your exercise routine every few months so that you don't plateau. If you were formerly morbidly obese and you've been able to lose weight through diet, exercise, and maybe even weight-loss surgery, you'll have to exercise for the rest of your life in order to guarantee that you remain at a healthy weight. If you don't exercise, then you'll have to go on such an extreme diet that you'll hardly be eating anything because your diet will be broken down to the "ninth macronutrient," making your chances of success slim to none. Combining routine exercise and moderate caloric intake is the only option for anyone who has formerly been morbidly obese.

In the initial stages of weight loss, dietary intake is the most important factor. Dr. Rogers states that a diet consisting of lean protein and non-starchy vegetables, with a small portion of fruit each day, is an ideal weight-loss diet. Rogers recommends eating four to six small meals throughout the day. If you are a non-surgical weight-loss patient, eating one meal a can be very detrimental to your weight-loss success. The reason for this is because eating once a day will slow your metabolism. The other problem is that if you eat only once a day, you will no doubt rationalize that you can eat more at your single daily meal because you haven't eaten all day. You'll compensate at that one meal and make up for all the calories you missed out on throughout the day. In addition, if you eat only one large meal, you are probably not going to feel all that great, which will also lead to inactivity. Eating one meal a day will set you up for failure in the long run.

If you are a surgical weight-loss patient, Rogers claims the most important thing is to stay hydrated and eat only when you're hungry. This being said, contrary to the non-surgical weight loss patient, a surgical patient can get away with eating one to two small meals, which, combined, may only total 300-600 calories a day. The reason for this is because surgical weight-loss patients have had their gastrointestinal system reconfigured and they do not digest food the same way the non-surgical patient does.

Dr. Rogers claims that in order to be successful, you have to change your lifestyle by following an exercise program and a well-balanced diet. You must create an eating plan that you enjoy. How you lose weight will help determine how you're going to be able to keep the weight off long term.

UNDERSTAND THE MEDICAL OPTIONS FOR WEIGHT LOSS

Dr. Rogers uses several different medical treatment options for weight loss. Pharmacotherapy or treating/preventing obesity with medications is one method she uses to facilitate weight loss. Caloric or macronutrient manipulation and exercise are other tactics. Rogers' manipulation of the macronutrient content depends on what an individual patient can tolerate in terms of a caloric deficit. If an individual's motivation is the weight reading on the scale and the person can handle deprivation, then Rogers puts the individual on a fairly aggressive weight-loss program. If a patient can't handle deprivation very well, then she explains to the individual that 1-2 lb of weight loss per week is okay. Depending on an individual's degree of obesity, Rogers may recommend weight-loss surgery.

Rogers says that putting a patient into ketosis is the best option for rapid weight loss. Ketosis is a form of macronutrient manipulation. How does ketosis contribute to weight loss and specifically fat loss? First, you must understand that your body depends on glucose, or glycogen, for its primary fuel source. Rogers explains that ketosis will occur if you deprive your body of glucose. Specifically, you need to limit the amount of starchy carbohydrates. This glucose deprivation will cause the body to start tapping into the stored glycogen in your liver. Your liver has about a three-day supply of stored glycogen in it. Once the body depletes the glycogen in the liver, it will begin to start using fat for fuel through a process called *beta oxidation*. When this occurs, the body is in a state of ketosis, meaning the body is forced to use stored fat as its primary fuel source. Two positive physiological effects to being in ketosis are (1) you're no longer hungry and (2) you'll have more energy. In combination, these two effects significantly help one's weight-loss efforts.

Rogers states that there are some contraindications to ketosis and that only a physician should put an individual into a state of ketosis. On the prescribed diet for inducing ketosis under a physician's supervision, a person can stay in ketosis for several months; however, due to the limited amount of fruits and vegetables one eats on this type of diet, it is very important to supplement the diet with micronutrients.

Some people want to know how many pounds a week is healthy weight loss. Dr. Rogers likes to think about a percentage of weight loss rather than pounds of weight lost. The reason for this is because the number of pounds a person can lose in one week really depends on how much total weight that particular person has to lose in the first place. So if one weighs 300 lb and loses 10 lb the first week, that's really only a 3-percent loss of one's total weight; this would be considered healthy weight loss. However, if one weighs 130 lb and loses 10 lb, this would equal a 13-percent loss of one's total weight in one week; Rogers doesn't recommend this rapid of weight loss for a person who weighs 130 lb to begin with. The other factor is whether or not you are losing the weight medically or surgically. If you are a surgical patient, you're going to lose weight much faster than a typical medical weight-loss patient.

REALIZE THAT ACCOUNTABILITY INCREASES SUCCESS

One must be accountable to oneself or someone else in order to foster success. In other words, you need to record what you are doing, constantly monitor your progress, and learn from your mistakes. If you can cognitively monitor what you eat and how active you are, you'll tend to be more successful. On the flip side, mindlessly eating without being aware of what you're doing will lead to disappointment and limited success or failure. One tool that is very beneficial is keeping a journal of your diet, exercise, and thoughts. Do this for one to two weeks and identify what things are contributing to weight loss or weight gain. Did you go out to eat five times last week and gain two pounds? Maybe the week before you ate really healthy and exercised four times for an hour each session and lost 3 lb. Can you understand what your obstacles were and when they occurred? Keeping track of your actions is very important. If you gained weight one week, it is important to be able to look back and identify the reasons you might have gained the weight. Learn from your mistakes and allow yourself to get back on track. Follow-up and accountability are important tools for success solutions if you are having trouble losing weight and keeping it off. People are motivated when they feel like they are achieving their goals and can see and measure their accomplishments.

Rogers claims that anyone can lose weight. She says if you are motivated, inquisitive, don't have a lot of distractions in your life, don't make excuses, are dedicated to improving your well-being, and make time for yourself, your chances of weight-loss success are high.

A BARIATRIC SURGEON'S PERSPECTIVE
BY DR. LLOYD STEGEMANN

PROFILE OF MM

MM is a 35-year-old female who came to me in 2005 to be evaluated for weight-loss surgery. At the time she weighed 305 lb and was experiencing many of the health problems that result from carrying an excessive amount of body weight. MM also felt incredibly fatigued and found it difficult to muster the energy to get through her daily routine. She subsequently underwent surgery, and at her most recent follow-up visit she had maintained a weight of 160 lb and reported that she felt "like a kid again."

PROFILE OF AS

AS is a 40-year-old female who also was evaluated by me for weight-loss surgery around the same time as MM. She weighed 295 lb at the time and also suffered from several weight-related medical problems. AS had surgery and, over the course of the next year, got down to a weight of 170 lb. However, at her most recent follow-up appointment AS had regained 50 lb and voiced her concern that she would "gain it all back."

Why is it that MM is able to maintain her weight loss while AS is struggling? Is there anything we can learn from their experiences? As a practicing weight-loss surgeon, I am often asked by patients, "What do I need to do to be successful with my weight loss?" I believe there are five principles that need to be learned and reinforced over time.

FIVE PRINCIPLES OF SUCCESSFUL WEIGHT LOSS

1. Weight Loss Surgery Is A Powerful Treatment For Obesity; It Is Not A Cure.

Is it possible for a patient to regain all of the weight they have lost after weight-loss surgery? Absolutely, positively, without a doubt, unequivocally. . . YES! The causes of obesity are complex, and currently many are not well understood. In addition, there probably isn't a *single* cause of obesity. Most likely there is a whole host of events that contribute to individuals' gaining excessive amounts of weight.

Weight-loss surgery is just one tool that can be used to treat obesity. However, like any tool, to maximize its efficacy, you have to learn how to use it properly.

There is *no* weight-loss operation available that a determined patient can't defeat if that is the person's goal. The successful patient understands this clearly and uses their weight-loss surgery as an opportunity to address the issues and habits that led to becoming obese.

Why can patients be successful with weight-loss surgery when they have failed so many times with conventional dieting? I believe the answer is that with weight-loss surgery, a patient can achieve two things: hunger control and food-volume control. By controlling these two key factors, a patient has an opportunity to start addressing other lifestyle issues.

2. Lifestyle = Weight.

I ask every patient that comes to me to be evaluated for surgery the same question: "Why do you think you struggle with your weight?" You would be amazed at the responses I get! Half of the time I get the answer "I really don't know." Other times it is "All my family struggles with their weight" or "My metabolism is slow." It is definitely a minority of the time that a patient will tell me "I have poor eating habits and I'm not as active as I need to be." I believe this is a *very* important point. After surgery, successful patients take ownership of their weight issues! Ultimately each of us decides what we put into our mouth, how we spend our time, and how we want to structure our lives. Our weight is simply a reflection of our lifestyle. If we lead a healthier lifestyle, we can achieve a healthier weight.

One of my favorite quotes is by Benjamin Franklin, who said, "The definition of insanity is doing the same thing over and over and expecting different results." This quote should become the mantra for every weight-loss surgery patient. If a patient does not recognize the lifestyle issues that got them to the point of needing weight-loss surgery, they will be unable to address these issues after surgery, and they will not be successful long term.

3. Failure To Plan Is Planning To Fail.

Figuring out what lifestyle issues need to be addressed is critical, but it is only half of the equation. The second step, which is much more challenging, is developing and implementing a plan to change these lifestyle issues. Another of my favorite quotes comes from Aristotle, who said, "We are what we repeatedly do. Excellence then, is not an act, but a habit."

Change is hard–period. There's no way around it. If it were easy, then no one would struggle to change. The hardest part of implementing change in your life is getting started. Author and playwright Juliene Berk put it aptly when she said, "Habits . . . the only reason they persist is that they are offering some satisfaction . . . You allow them to persist by not seeking any other, better form of satisfying the same needs. Every habit, good or bad, is acquired and learned in the same way—by finding that it is a means of satisfaction." This is especially true when it comes to behavioral changes that are vital to long-term success. Why am I eating? Am I eating because I am happy, sad, angry, stressed, etc., or because I am hungry? The emotions that lead to overeating and poor eating habits are real, but to be successful in changing bad habits, one needs to find ways to deal with these emotions without using food.

Changing habits does not come easy, nor does it come quickly. Noted author Mark Twain knew this when he wrote, "A habit cannot be tossed out the window; it must be coaxed down the stairs a step at a time." Patients often set themselves up for frustration and failure by trying to change a habit quickly. I see this all the time when it comes to exercise. Prior to surgery, most of my patients participated in very little physical activity. After surgery they understand how important activity is, so they jump in with both feet and work out way too hard! This often leads to soreness, frustration, and occasionally injury. Change is much easier to accept if it is made gradually. This involves setting a goal and then developing specific steps to get you there.

4. The Road To A Healthier Life Has Many Curves And Some Road Hazards.

For some people, the road to health is a very straight road indeed. After surgery they adapt to all of the necessary lifestyle changes quickly and just never look back. They "get it," and for these lucky few, food is no longer an issue but rather a necessity. For the majority of people, however, the road looks more like zigzagging Lombard Street (a street in San Francisco famous for having a steep, one-block section consisting of tight hairpin turns)! They are on track and then go sideways, only to recover and get back on track again. Successful patients recognize when they are approaching a curve (weight regain or prolonged plateau) and they slow down so they don't lose control! In slowing down they either make an appointment with their surgeon or physician in their weight loss program, go to a support group, or review their "owner's manual" and refresh themselves on their program's "rules of the road." Hopefully, they will do all three! A weight-loss patient shouldn't expect to get it right 100 percent of the time, and if they hold themselves to this unrealistic expectation, they are likely to get frustrated and give up. The truth of the matter is that if they are getting it right 70 percent of the time, they are likely to maintain their weight loss over time. You see, there is no *one* meal that will sabotage weight loss. It is the 10 meals before and 10 meals after that *one* meal that make a *much* bigger difference in successfully losing weight long term!

Many patients think that once they reach their goal weight they can stop and relax. Nothing could be further from the truth! I think this misconception is a holdover from the "diet mentality" that many patients have before surgery. You see, diets are temporary interventions designed to be done for a short period of time until a certain weight goal is obtained and then they are stopped. I often tell my patients "After surgery, I won't put you on a diet; I'll put you on a lifestyle." Our weight is a reflection of our lifestyle, and if patients return to their old lifestyle, they will return to their old weight!

5. FAILURE IS NOT AN OPTION.

The successful patient has a steadfast resolve to succeed in their weight-loss journey, while the unsuccessful patient expects failure. I believe this also is a holdover from the "diet mentality." Most patients experienced yo-yo dieting prior to opting for weight-loss surgery: For example, a patient may lose 5 lb on a diet and then gain back 7 lb, lose another 10 lb and then gain 15 lb, as they "dieted" their way to morbid obesity. Unfortunately, some patients retain this mentality after surgery. At the first sign of a set back, unsuccessful patients tell themselves, "I knew it wouldn't work for me." When they have a setback, successful patients, on the other hand, tell themselves, "HELL no, I'm not going back!" Coach Vince Lombardi hit the nail on the head when he said, "The difference between a successful person and others is not a lack of strength, not a lack of knowledge, but rather a lack of will." The successful patient says, "I will *not* fail."

You see, each weight-loss surgery patient is given a second chance at the time of surgery—a do-over of sorts. The real question is what they will do with this second chance. Will they be like MM and learn from their previous mistakes and take the opportunity to lead a healthier life? Or will they be like AS and return to the old habits that got them to the point at which they needed weight-loss surgery? The fact that you are reading this book is a good sign you are in the former group. I wish you much success on your weight-loss journey.

A PSYCHOLOGIST'S PERSPECTIVE

This section identifies what it takes from a psychologist's perspective to be successful in one's attempts to lose weight. Everything outlined in this chapter was taken from an interview the author conducted with Dr. Edward Wilks on January 9, 2008. Dr. Wilks is a licensed psychologist as well as a licensed marriage and family therapist. He has been doing clinical work for 22 years. Most recently he's been practicing psychological intervention for physical and medical conditions. For the past two years he has done psychological counseling with individuals trying to lose weight. He feels that the better people understand their conditions as well as the remedies and treatment for these conditions, the more effective the result.

Emotional and mental factors significantly influence one's ability to be successful with weight loss. Some people have self-destructive habits or skills that thwart their weight-loss efforts, while others have healthy habits and skills that foster successful weight loss. Many overweight and obese individuals overeat in order to alleviate moods and unwelcome emotional states. It is paramount for one to recognize the actions, feelings, and thoughts that trigger emotional eating. If you are able to recognize what is about to happen, you'll be capable of taking action to prevent unhealthy habits.

One of the tools used in psychology is called *cognitive behavioral therapy*. This has to do with helping an individual identify and transform the meaning we assign to events, situations, and experiences. Ask yourself these two questions: What is my belief about my current weight or size? What kind of beliefs do I have about the potential for change? Now, consider your answers to these questions relative to the two distinct styles of cognitive behavior or thinking outlined below—successful thinking and unsuccessful thinking.

- *Successful thinking*
  "I need to start watching what I eat."
  "I'm going to start an exercise program."
  "I shouldn't be so hard on myself."

"I'm ready to make a change for me."
"I want to do the things I used to do."
"I am fat because I've made some poor choices in my eating selection."
"I'm not going to let things get in the way of my goals."

- *Unsuccessful thinking*
"This is how my whole family is, we're all overweight."
"I'm fat because of my mother"
"I've never been able to be physically active."
"I'm never going to be able to lose weight"
"I am overweight because of a surgery I had five years ago."
"I'm fat because of my job."
"I'm not meant to be thin."
"I don't think I'll be able to do the things I need to do to lose weight."

The meaning you assign to situations, events, and experiences makes all the difference. How you think and how you regard yourself makes a big difference in your overall success. If you are optimistic and aware that you can make a difference, you'll have a better chance of losing weight.

COGNITIVE DISTORTIONS

Dr. Wilks initially interviews people to see what type of cognitive-style thinking they've been using. He refers to a list of cognitive distortions developed by David D. Burns to identify areas in which people may have been creating difficulties for themselves without realizing it [1]. Burns believes that cognitive distortions cause many, if not all, of a person's depressed states. See the following table, which defines the various types of cognitive distortions identified by Burns.

Cognitive Distortions

All-or-nothing thinking	You see things in black and white categories. If your performance falls short of perfect, you see yourself as a total failure.
Overgeneralization	You see a single negative event as a never-ending pattern of defeat.

Mental filtering	You pick out a single negative detail and dwell on it exclusively so that your vision of all reality becomes darkened, like the drop of ink that discolors an entire beaker of water.
Disqualifying the positive	You reject positive experiences by insisting they "don't count" for some reason or another. In this way, you can maintain a negative belief that is contradicted by your everyday experiences.
Jumping to conclusions	You make a negative interpretation even though there are no definite facts that convincingly support your conclusion.
Mind reading	You arbitrarily conclude that someone is reacting negatively to you, and you don't bother to check this out.
The fortune-teller error	You anticipate that things will turn out badly, and you feel convinced that your prediction is an already established fact.
Magnification or minimization	You exaggerate the importance of things (such as your goof-up or someone else's achievements) or you inappropriately shrink things until they appear tiny (your own desirable qualities or the other fellow's imperfections). This is also called the *binocular trick*.
Emotional reasoning	You assume that your negative emotions necessarily reflect the way things really are. "I feel it therefore it must be true."

"Should" statements	You try to motivate yourself with "shoulds" and "shouldn'ts" as if you had to be whipped and punished before you could be expected to do anything. "Musts" and "oughts" are also offenders. The emotional consequence is guilt. When you direct "should" statements toward others you feel anger, frustration, and resentment.
Labeling and mislabeling	This is an extreme form of overgeneralization. Instead of describing your error, you attach a negative label to yourself: "I'm a loser." When someone else's behavior rubs you the wrong way, you attach a negative label to him: "He's a loser." Mislabeling involves describing an event with language that is highly colored and emotionally loaded.
Personalization	You see yourself as the cause of some negative external event, which in fact you were not primarily responsible for.

Source: From *The Feel Good Handbook* [1].

Dr. Wilks explains some of David Burn's cognitive-thinking characteristics in more detail as they relate to one's ability to be successful in losing weight.

ALL-OR-NOTHING THINKING

All-or-nothing thinking can help determine whether one will be successful or not in their weight-loss efforts. All-or-nothing thinking is a cognitive distortion; essentially it is thinking that is "out of shape," not correct, or dismorphic. People who think like this tend to see the world in polar opposites or extremes, with essentially no middle ground: Something is true or false, wrong or right, black or white. They have an "if I can't do this I'm just going to quit" mentality.

Dr. Wilks often refers to this type of thinking as *distressed thinking*, a form of inefficient, skewed cognition characterized by thinking in extremes. For example, "I need to quit my job" or "I have to get out of this marriage." An example of extreme distressed thinking is "I want to die." This style of thinking misses all the gradations in between, thus omitting all of the possibilities in the middle. All-or-nothing thinkers can become very pessimistic when encountered by any setback and they often struggle in their weight-loss attempts. If they cheat on their diet, they may decide to quit the whole weight-loss thing all together. Or maybe they weren't able to lose 10 lb in one month, so they just stop trying to lose weight. Distressed thinking is often why people are unsuccessful in losing weight. Distressed thinkers tend to lose their motivation all together and quit their weight-loss program.

Another problem with this style of thinking is that if and when distressed thinkers do meet one of their goals, what next? Do they just stop after meeting a weight-loss goal or finishing a race? Are they capable of continuing to follow their new healthy habits, or do they fall back into old habits and gain back the weight they've lost? You can't live your life at the finish line; you must move on. The problem with distressed thinkers is that they tend to establish a static, rigid goal for completion, and if they do not complete or achieve it fairly easily or quickly, they tend to believe they've failed. Remember, you can't live at the finish line, nor can you live at the starting line. What happens along the way is very important, and you always need to move forward.

An all-or-nothing thinker is likely to "bail out" on their goals in a way that is out of proportion to what setback(s) have actually happened. The ability to get back on track without feeling self-defeated is very important. Dr. Wilks uses driving a car as a metaphor to help people realize what they are doing when they use all-or-nothing thinking: If you are driving a car and all of a sudden you hear and feel a vibration, what just happened? Maybe you drove onto the shoulder or possibly crossed the middle of the road and the vibration you feel is caused by the road reflectors or the grooved section on the side of the road that you just drove on. Wilks says you need to refer to these road reflectors or grooved areas as "road reminders." When people drive onto these "road reminders," they've just received a message telling them to get back in the "middle of the road." Now you have awareness of where you are and the vibration has given you feedback to get back on the road. So ask yourself this question: What have you done when you've encountered "road reminders"? I bet you answered something like this: "Well I better pay more attention to the road" or "I better pay attention and get back in my lane of the road." The road reminders tell you to get back on the road and pay closer attention. People generally don't stop the car altogether on the side of the road and say, "Well my goodness, I need to stop what I'm doing because I simply can't drive anymore."

Wilks encourages people to use the driving-a-car analogy to help people attempting to lose weight stay focused on what they are trying to do. For example, if you ate five cookies over the weekend, you "drove over five road reminders." You just have to understand that these cookies are your road reminders. You drove a little off the road this weekend and now you need to pay closer attention and get back on track with your diet. Your lapse doesn't mean that you have to quit your diet. Never throw in the towel because of a setback.

LABELING OR MISLABELING

Self-labeling—or mislabeling—involves how you regard yourself. If you make the remark "I'm a failure" or "I'm a loser," you've just labeled yourself a failure or loser and are reinforcing this negative self-labeling in your mind. If you use an adjective to label yourself, it should have a positive, affirming connotation. A positive label would be "I am a learner." Using the example mentioned above, positive labeling would be that you had a *learning* experience when you ate five cookies over the weekend; you took a message and learned from it by correcting future actions or performance. The problem with becoming a learner is that when a learning task that is daunting or challenging is encountered, at first, many people may avoid the situation. Often, people are afraid to fail or feel ashamed because they might fail. This can cause them to avoid taking action. This type of thinking—fear of failure—can talk us into staying on the sidelines.

Sometimes we avoid new (and positive) situations because we feel awkward. Let's start to think about awkwardness in a new way. Many of us think of awkwardness as something that should be avoided. If one doesn't feel comfortable, it's usually because the situation is unfamiliar, and chances are one will avoid it. This type of thinking is a recipe for sameness. If the goal is weight loss and you stay the same, you won't be successful in your weight-loss goals because you'll be unable to change the habits that have created the being that you are today—carrying around excess body fat. Instead of avoiding awkwardness, let's practice *embracing* it instead. Awkwardness is actually a symptom that you're about to learn something new and different, not a message that the situation is dangerous and should be avoided. Learning to read the signals correctly can help us progress. People that are "allergic" to feeling awkward are not likely to learn new things this leaves them with what they already know. Learners change, adapt, and grow. Learners are able to receive feedback from situations and get back on track with their weight-loss goals: "I've learned what it is like to eat and be with my family despite being on this new diet"; I've learned how to say no to the excess food that has been a consistent theme in my family"; "I've learned how to push back."

MENTAL FILTERING

Dr. Wilks leads different support groups on a regular basis, and sometimes he'll throw out this question to the crowd: "How would everyone like a recipe for misery?" Not too many people are interested in finding out more, and there are few affirmative responses. Then he asks, "How about a recipe for success?" Most people want to know a recipe for success, so this question elicits several "yeses." However, the truth is that many people create recipes for misery or success in their minds. Let's think about filters—they hang onto some things and let go of others. Think of common filters around the house, a dryer filter, an air conditioner filter, an oil filter in your car. They are full of the impurities that we're trying to eliminate. How would you like to hang out with impurities all day? A negative mental filter is just that: a collection of negative memories and beliefs that we've hung onto while the positive memories and beliefs flowed on through. It's time we cleaned out the "dryer lint" in our heads, all those thoughts like, "I'm a failure," "I can't do this," "I'll only be successful when I meet my goal weight," "I'll never be able to find a man that is attracted to me," "Men don't notice me," and "Women don't notice me." Once we've cleaned out our filter, let's install a positive filter in its place, one that keeps only positive thoughts, "I'm a learner," "I will lose 20 lb," "I can be physically active," and "I want to overcome my obstacles." Managing our mental filters is a major key to success.

Another form of destructive reasoning is called the *fortune-teller error*. You anticipate that things will turn out badly and you're convinced that your predictions will come true. An example of this kind of thought process would be convincing yourself that you're never going to be able to lose weight. You tell yourself this over and over again and feel defeated to the point that you never really try to lose weight because you are convinced that you can't lose any weight. This is destructive reasoning and will definitely hinder your success in trying to lose weight because you've already convinced yourself that you aren't able to lose weight. Another example of fortune-teller error would be telling yourself that you can't get promoted. Every time something bad happens at work you feel as if those things were going to happen regardless because you can't seem to do anything right and you're convinced that you'll never get promoted because bad things continue to happen to you.

EMOTIONAL REASONING

Dr. Wilks says we're always creating fiction in our heads. In our minds we all have our own personal Stephen King; he constantly writes personalized horror stories derived from our ideas, thoughts, worst fears, and insecurities. These stories stem from the insecurities, problems, and traumas that have happened to us throughout our lives. Our personal author starts writing things like, "The reason you can't do this is because you're a loser," "You don't have the ability to be successful," "You've tried weight loss diets before and it's never worked; you've failed at every attempt," or "The reason he didn't call you back is because you're not good enough for him." All of these negative thoughts may cause you to start believing this mental feedback of your own creation, and you may begin to think of yourself in very critical ways. In fact, some tasks you won't even overtake anymore because they foster these thoughts and feelings of being defeated due to your insecurities.

Emotional reasoning is a classic way of thinking: I feel it; therefore, it must be true. We all tend to experience this kind of distressed thinking at times. In this way we create our own problems for ourselves: It isn't necessarily the world that has caused a particular problem, but rather how we've interpreted the world and our experiences in it.

LEARNED HELPLESSNESS

Do people that have more stable mental or psychological states have a better chance to be successful in their weight-loss efforts? Martin E. P. Seligman did some studies on what he called *learned helplessness*, a theory of depression [2]. His studies showed that a helpless, depressed state can be created by exposing an individual to repeated trauma to a point at which the individual stops attempting to avoid or escape the trauma—in other words, acts helpless. The investigators conducting the studies first experimented with dogs. They put the dogs in cages, and whenever a dog tried to leave its cage, the investigators would sound a bell or horn and then shock the dog through the floor. Eventually, the dogs became passive and lost motivation to try leaving their cages. The dogs became so passive that when they'd hear the bell, they wouldn't even move or do anything because they had lost all motivation to try leaving or escaping from the cage. The dogs in this study were essentially trained to act helpless. Even when the investigators put the dogs in different cages in which the dogs had a way to get out and the door was accessible and easy to push open, they still didn't try to leave their cages. They felt helpless and depressed due to the learned behavior stemming from how they'd been trained.

In this same study, the investigators put another group of dogs that had never been trained to be depressed or helpless in a cage where they would get shocked after the horn or bell sounded. When the horn sounded, these dogs would get out of the cage before they were shocked. Finally, they put the two different groups of dogs together in the same cage: the group that had been trained to be helpless and the group that wasn't trained to be helpless. After the trained-to-act helpless dogs saw how the untrained dogs escaped the cage, the former followed the lead of the latter and escaped the cage: They learned from the other group of dogs to leave the cage. They learned that in this new situation they could do something to escape the trauma and changed their behavior.

Dr. Wilks said a similar study was done with rats to determine how long a rat will swim before it gives up? The ones that had been trained to be helpless victims gave up long before the other rats. The rats that had not been trained to be helpless and were equally fit and strong out swam the helpless rats.

This all correlates to self-efficacy. Self-efficacy is an understanding that what you do makes a difference—in other words, that there is value and benefit to the decisions and actions you are taking. For example, eating a salad instead of fried chicken really does make a difference in terms of weight control and overall health. The sooner you realize that your actions directly affect your success, the sooner you'll build self-confidence. Self-confidence and self-efficacy go hand in hand.

SUPPORT STRUCTURES

Family, friends, and strong support systems are important. People who have social support, in particular family and friends, tend to be more successful in their weight-loss efforts; however, the key is *using* this social support. Some people have it but don't use it. Attending support groups is another way for people to talk about their problems and solutions. Individuals in the group learn that they are not alone in experiencing and facing problems and resolving them. When they see that another person has changed, they can believe that they, too, can change. Social support is essentially what Oprah and Dr. Phil have done on their talk shows: People learn from others' experiences through a televised support group. All types of learning through various support systems are referred to as social learning. An individual can learn from others' struggles and triumphs.

Websites are other great ways to access social support. *ObesityHelp.com* provides thousands of scenarios that empower people to learn, share, and connect with others who have faced similar problems or situations. Their stories of how they dealt with particular problems or situations often have a more profound impact than guidance from a professional. It is usually invaluable to hear from someone that doesn't have a professional license or vested interest (e.g., a professional fee) and has personally experienced similar situations.

POSITIVE PSYCHOLOGY AND BEING SUCCESSFUL

One of the books Seligman wrote is titled *Learned Optimism*. In this book, he explains how an individual can develop skills in order to be more optimistic [2]. Let's say you've been taught to act like a victim due to previous experiences. You have to unlearn this behavior and relearn how to be optimistic through other positive experiences that happen in your life.

In order to be successful, you must learn how to overcome negative thinking. Realizing that you have negative thinking is the first step. If you realize that you are starting to think negatively, you can catch yourself and avoid the downward spiral. Dr. Wilks encourages people to be aware of what they're feeling and what they're telling themselves (their internal monologue). Healthy people are self-aware people; they are aware what specific thoughts and beliefs are influencing them. Consider this example: Your husband makes a negative comment about your weight-loss efforts. You can let that derail you, or you can say to yourself,

"Here is my husband giving me these messages, and I think my husband is feeling challenged about me changing my life because he's not used to this change." You can decide you're not going to allow him to "put one over" on you like he may have done in the past: You're not going to let him "talk you out" of doing things that will allow you to achieve your weight-loss goals. Your response to your husband might be "Look honey, thanks for your concern, but I'm going to the gym now." Try to neutralize your comments so that they aren't negative, abrasive, or self-destructive. Use benevolent and caring language rather than sarcasm, defensiveness, or verbal aggression to react to your husband's comments. Learning how to respond to these types of negative comments will keep you focused on your goal to lose weight and help prevent being thrown off balance.

TOWARD AND AWAY-FROM GOALS

Goals are ideas or intentions about how you want your future to be—or not be. Goals can be expressed in two ways: (1) *toward goals*, goals you want to achieve, accomplish, or experience or (2) *away-from goals*, the things you want to avoid, don't care to experience, or have to stop from happening.

TOWARD GOALS MIGHT BE SOMETHING LIKE THIS:

- "I can't wait to lose 100 lb and fit into that beautiful black sequined dress I saw in the department store last week. I want to get down to a size 10 and then I can wear that beautiful dress to the Christmas party next year."
- "When I get down to my goal weight, I'm going to be able to play with my grandchildren. I'll chase them around the yard and play catch with them. I want to show them what Grandpa can do."
- "Once I get in better shape, I'm going to be able to play a round of golf with the guys and they won't have to stop one time to wait on me. I'll also be able to shave 10 strokes off my 18-hole score."

Toward goals allow you to visualize yourself enjoying positive experiences because of the weight you want to lose. Thoughts of "Yes, I am getting closer and closer to my goals and each day I am moving forward toward my destiny."

Other people have goals that include a long list of what they don't want. These types of goals might be something like this:

- "I don't want to have diabetes."
- "I don't want to have heart disease or die from a heart attack."
- "I don't want to take blood pressure medication."
- "I don't want to have to take insulin injections every day."
- "I don't want to have knee surgery."
- "I don't want to have high cholesterol."

All of these are away-from goals: things you want to avoid. The problem with these goals is that people think about things in terms of mental images. So, if I told you to think about a car that is not red, chances are that you would think about a red car. This is how the human brain processes things; the subconscious takes out the "not." We think of what it *is* versus what it is *not*, and this is driven by our subconscious brain. So, if all of your goals are away-from goals, you may not be extremely motivated because your brain will process negatives like diabetes, high cholesterol, high blood pressure, or heart attack, all of your greatest fears. These fears may motivate you to exercise and eat healthy to a degree, but how long is your motivation going to last and what are your goals? If you keep looking back at all of the things you don't want, you can't properly focus on your goals—what you *do* want. It's like driving your car and looking in the rearview mirror the entire time you're driving: You know exactly where you are *not* going. If you are more aware and focused on where you're not, or where you're trying to get away from, you might encounter some problems: If you are driving your car while only looking at where you've been, you might end up in someone's lawn, in the ditch, or crash into a wall. Dr. Wilks encourages people to have a mental image and be aware of where they are going or where they want to be. It is good to be aware of where you've been and also understand your fears, but you have to know where you are going. Fears may prod you to move forward a little bit, but you must plug into your motivation and positive energy, determination, and certainty about achieving your goals. This will give you a "yes, I'm moving in the right direction" mindset, a characteristic of successful people. You are able to link specific routine habits and behaviors with progress toward your goals.

SELF-ACTUALIZATION

Once you get to this point of success, how do you stay on track to either maintain your weight, if you've achieved your goal weight, or continue to lose weight to meet the next goal? If you see yourself moving in the direction of your toward goals and are also aware of your away-from goals, you will continue to be on the path of success. You will also come to the self-actualization of who you really want to be. You've changed your identity; you no longer think of yourself as unhealthy and physically unfit. Now, you see yourself as a healthy, exercising-type person. You actually enjoy your new healthy habits and have progressed to the point that you practice them automatically. You no longer have to constantly think about making the best decision for continued weight-loss success.

In order to stay on track, however, a person has to recalibrate, that is, identify what is "delicious" about being at this new goal weight: Now you can enjoy daily activities: You're able to walk up a flight of stairs; you can fit in a normal-sized chair; you're able to bend over and tie your shoes; you can paint your toenails; you can walk a mile in 15 minutes; etc.

INTERPRETING SETBACKS

The ability to get back on track without feeling self-defeated is very important. You have to be able to recognize setbacks and react accordingly in a way similar to how running over road reflectors ("road reminders") while driving helps you realize when you're getting off track. Use this driving-a-car analogy, as outlined in the all-or-nothing section, to help you stay focused on what you're trying to accomplish—to lose weight! If you slipped up and ate five cookies over the weekend, understand that you "drove a little off the road" over the weekend and now you need to pay closer attention and get back on track with your diet.

Even successful people can experience setbacks, but they know how to interpret them in a way that is not self-defeating so that the setbacks do not derail them from their path of success. They understand that setbacks are information, and they can confidently react to them. Maybe you ate too much when you went out to dinner last night with a group of friends and felt very uncomfortable afterward. You realize that this feeling is information in that it empowers you to make better decisions when eating out next time. So the next time you go out to eat with your friends, you see everyone else ordering heavy fried foods, but you make the decision to order grilled chicken with vegetables. You're okay with your friends' eating less healthy food and very satisfied with your decision to order a healthy entrée.

THE BIG PROBLEM: EATING WHEN YOU ARE NOT HUNGRY

Eating when you are not hungry is one of the biggest problems for people who struggle with controlling their weight. Overweight to obese individuals tend to be emotional eaters: They eat when they are depressed, happy, or bored. Eating when you're bored is a classic problem; you eat because you needed something to do. What tactics can you use to fill the emotional need to eat? The first step is to realize when you're feeling hungry but that the feeling is coming from your head, not your stomach. Hunger should come from visceral, physical feelings, not mental or emotional feelings.

If you are eating because you're bored, think of the opposite of boredom. The opposite of boredom is having something to do, right? That might be part of the picture, but it's not the whole picture and not necessarily a very clear picture. Sometimes you're eating not simply for a lack of something to do. The last time you ate when you weren't actually hungry you were probably doing something, for example, working on the computer or watching television. It wasn't the fact that you weren't doing something; rather, it was a lack of something *fun* to do. Food is something that is available, affordable, legal, won't reject you, and provides immediate gratification. Food is fun because it satisfies your need to feel better quickly. Many people who are angry, lonely, hurt, sad, stressed, or anxious turn to consumption of food in the refrigerator to alleviate these negative emotions. Before long, they may find themselves eating to resolve every unwelcome feeling.

If you find yourself in this vicious cycle, it is time to find something else that is available, affordable, legal, and won't "turn you down." Instead of giving in to your compulsion to eat, how about reading a book, getting on the computer, playing the guitar, painting, or going for a walk? Or maybe you should chew a piece of sugar free gum or drink some water. The point is to choose something that will allow you to expend your energy on a healthy alternative. Choose activities that will not foster the desire or compulsion to eat. If you do have these feelings, be consciously aware of them so you can resist them.

Be aware that if you feel like eating when you're not hungry, it is not a good idea to simply say to yourself, "Well, okay, I just won't eat." This would mean giving up what you use to comfort yourself and not replacing it with something else comforting or rewarding, thus setting yourself up for failure.

RECYCLING

Interestingly, a lot of people who gain weight are hoarders. They hang onto a lot of things and let things accumulate as if they may need all of these things someday. Sometimes, people hoard things out of a fear of scarcity; they collect too much stuff because they feel that the world has deprived them of things. They can't waste any food because "there are people starving in Africa." They eat as much as possible at a buffet because they want to get their money's worth. Or maybe, their parents taught them never to waste food, so they always clean their plate.

If you keep more than you're willing to let go of even if you don't need it, you are hording things, and no doubt you also hang onto fears, past experiences, resentments, and other negative emotions. It is time to let go! Letting go of things can be very liberating. In fact, some say that getting rid of clutter is an excellent weight-loss strategy. Getting more organized and cleaning things out makes many people feel energized. You may be one of these people—you may become more energetic, focused, and efficient if you've been able to get rid of things you don't need.

Some people have clothes in three different sizes because they fear they might need them later. People like this think, "Sure I lost 10 lb, but I might gain it back, so I need to hang on to the larger sizes." People horde things because of hypothetical ("what if") scenarios: "I might need this if . . ." If you haven't used or needed it in the past year, you probably don't need it at all, so get rid of it. Recycle it: Give it to someone who will use it. It will make you feel better. Keep the *memory* of that jacket you never wear anymore and get rid of the jacket itself. By recycling, you can give something away and feel good about it. You want to feel light, not heavy, so give it away. You don't need all of the things that are weighing you down. You become stagnant if you horde things and never let go. Don't be fearful of letting go; it can be a wonderful experience and lead to moving forward in achieving your weight-loss goals. You can think of losing weight as recycling—you are getting rid of the excess weight you don't want or need anymore. You need enough fuel (food) to survive and be active, but you do not need an excessive amount of food that will put fat on your body. So, next time you lay eyes on an awesome-looking donut, savor the thought of how it would taste but pass it by.

You may be thinking that some people might not want what you have to give away. How do you recycle toxic waste like bitterness, anger, resentment, or excess weight? First, you need to neutralize them, similar to how a sewage plant recycles sludge. Some sewage plants can recycle sewage into drinking water through a process that involves a whole lot of neutralization. Something that was once toxic can be made pure enough to drink; this is turning a bad thing into something wonderful. You can do similar things with toxic emotions. Take bitterness and turn it into positive action or a positive influence. For example, if you were abused as a child, use your toxic feelings about this experience to create a support system for abused children. Allow others to feel loved and not feel alone. How about anger? Anger can be very powerful in a positive way if it is properly channeled. In fact, some people *have* to get angry in order to make a change. Are you angry about all of the weight that you're carrying around? Are you angry that you can't get that promotion due to your weight? Channel that anger into fighting the fat. Utilize the "anger" energy and start losing weight.

SELF-PARENTING

Be kind to yourself. Learn how to treat yourself with good parenting skills. Treat yourself like a nurturing parent when you most need support and encouragement. Someone who is self-parenting is a successful adult. To be self-parenting is a great gift and a key to inner strength and resilience: Reward yourself for achieving your accomplishments. Celebrate the small victories on your way to the ultimate victory of getting to your goal weight and also comfort yourself when you are hurting. Give yourself what you need, and when you need support from a friend or family member, pick up the phone or ask to get together to tap into the support that is available to you.

POSITIVE PSYCHOLOGY THROUGH EXERCISE

Physical activity has a very positive mental effect on people. Understand that exercise is going to help you do the things you want to do. Don't think too hard about the actual physical act of exercising; you may not thoroughly enjoy physical activity. However, understand that exercise will allow you to do more things that will positively impact your psychological state. Exercise is a great stress reliever, and for many of us, this is paramount to ensure negative thoughts do not pile up.

Get rid of the "toxins" and embrace the new, positive and physically active you. You'll feel better about yourself, be able to handle stress, and lose weight!

In closing, your psychological state, from how you think to how you react to situations, will play a very important role in your overall success or failure with regard to weight loss. As the saying goes, "You control your own destiny." Your emotional state will help determine your success. Allow yourself to be positive, accept a challenge or "hiccup" in your program as feedback to help you get back on track, and surround yourself with a strong support group.

REFERENCES

1. Burns, David D. *The Feel Good Handbook.* New York: Penguin, 1999.
2. Seligman, Martin EP. *Learned Optimism: How to Change Your Mind and Your Life.* New York: Random House, 2006.

Chapter 10
Client Testimonials

Rx Fitness for Weight Loss: The Medically Sound Solution to Get Fit and Save Your Life

MICHELLE TALLON

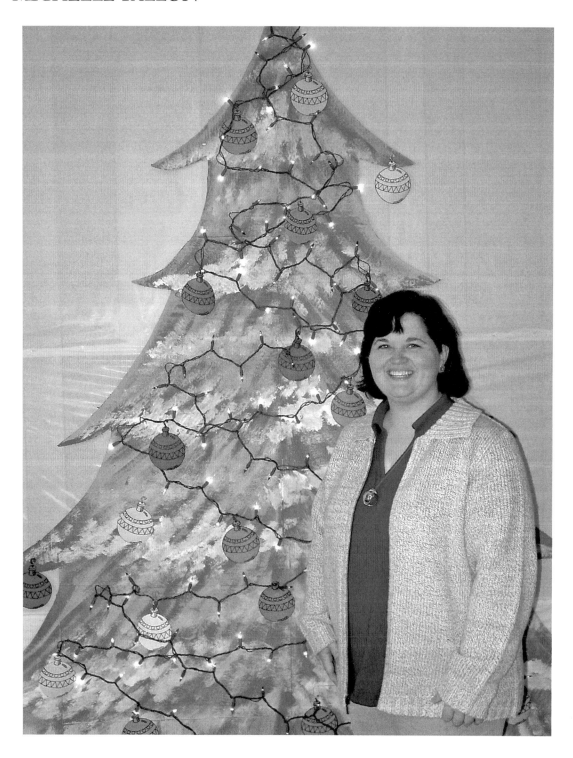

Client Testimonials

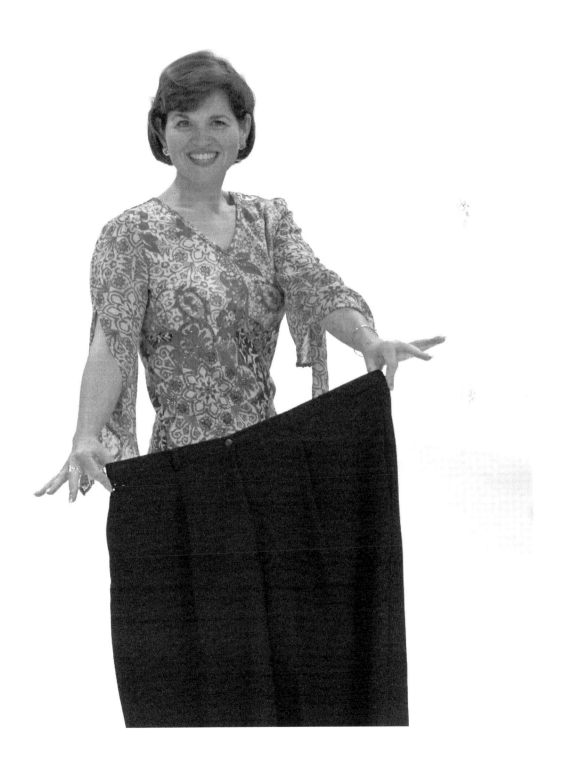

Rx Fitness for Weight Loss: The Medically Sound Solution to Get Fit and Save Your Life

I had been overweight my entire life; in fact, most of my family is overweight. I remember that when I was young, both of my parents were suffering through many weight-related health problems. When my mother passed away, I decided that I wanted to be healthier so I would not have to suffer through some of the same problems. I weighed 188 lb when I made a decision to see a doctor who specialized in weight loss and to get serious about making a change in my life. After my initial consultation, which included routine lab work, I discovered that I had high blood pressure, high cholesterol, and was classified as obese. All of these problems put me at high risk for major medical problems, including diabetes and heart disease. Although I had always been heavy, I had never really seen myself as heavy or obese. However, facts are facts, and it was time to face reality.

The doctor suggested that I first see a nutritionist to discuss a healthy eating plan. I took the advice and met with the nutritionist. We discussed many issues, and she worked with me to understand what I liked to eat versus what I should be eating. I slowly changed my dietary habits and started eating three healthy, moderately sized meals a day plus one healthy snack. Most important, I gave up drinking regular soda. The nutritionist made me aware that one regular soda contributed an extra 150 calories a day that I didn't really need. For the next four months I met regularly with the nutritionist and religiously followed my dietary plan, I was doing great—I was losing weight and receiving compliments almost everywhere I went. However, at my six-month checkup with the doctor, I found out that my blood pressure and cholesterol were still in unhealthy ranges; in fact my HDL (the "good" cholesterol) was very low. I didn't understand why these were still problematic, since I'd lost weight and was feeling pretty good. I asked the doctor why, and she gave me a long detailed answer that basically boiled down to not getting enough exercise. Yep, I needed to exercise. In fact, the last time I had exercised was in physical education class back in high school. I had never really cared for physical activity, but since my current state of health was not optimal, I decided to give it a whirl. I recruited the help of my best friend, and together we decided to sign up for personal training sessions. At this point I met Julia Karlstad.

I was excited that Julia was going to be my personal trainer because she held both Bachelor of Science and Master of Education degrees in exercise science. She also had many fitness certifications and was both enthusiastic and encouraging in her approach to training. Julia began my program by assessing my individual fitness abilities. I completed several tests, including both a resting metabolic rate assessment and a VO2 indirect calorimetry assessment. The results were what I expected: My physical fitness fell in the "below average" category. Although I was somewhat depressed and discouraged, Julia explained to me how we, together, were going to change this fitness level. Not only did Julia motivate me through physical training, but she also discussed the importance of healthy eating. The one thing that Julia said that sticks with me today is that exercise is the one thing that can minimize the occasional slip-up. In other words, if you eat a little too much or eat the wrong thing now and then, exercise helps combat the negative results of doing so. Now, this doesn't mean you can slip up all the time, but exercise acts like insurance to prevent you from getting too far off track. Exercise helps your body burn fat and increases your total caloric burn for one day. Julia was there to motivate and coach me toward my wellness and weight-loss goals. She made every appointment fun; actually, her motto is "Exercise can be fun." She was energetic and motivating and always encouraged me to perform at my maximum capacity. The few times that I hit a plateau, Julia was there to re-evaluate my exercise prescription and adjust it as needed.

When I went to see the doctor a few months later, I received great news . . . in fact I was very surprised. Not only were my blood pressure and cholesterol within the normal range, but so was my body mass index (BMI). I got these results through exercise and diet, and I would have never achieved them through diet alone. Today I weigh 123 lb and my BMI is 23.2, well within the normal range. I lost a total of 65 pounds. Julia taught me that although I may achieve a healthy weight, exercise would always need to be a part of my life, not just a stint to get me to a weight goal—that is, exercise needed to be a permanent part of my lifestyle. If I wanted to stay at my healthy weight, I'd need to continue my physical activity. Although I'm not a big fan of exercise, I really enjoy the benefits of it, and that's enough to keep me moving. Overall fitness has greatly improved the quality of my life. I not only feel and look better, but I'm much healthier!

Rx Fitness for Weight Loss: The Medically Sound Solution to Get Fit and Save Your Life

KIM OERKFITZ

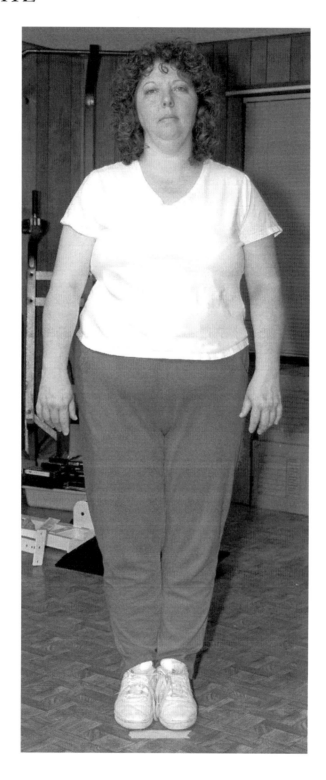

Client Testimonials

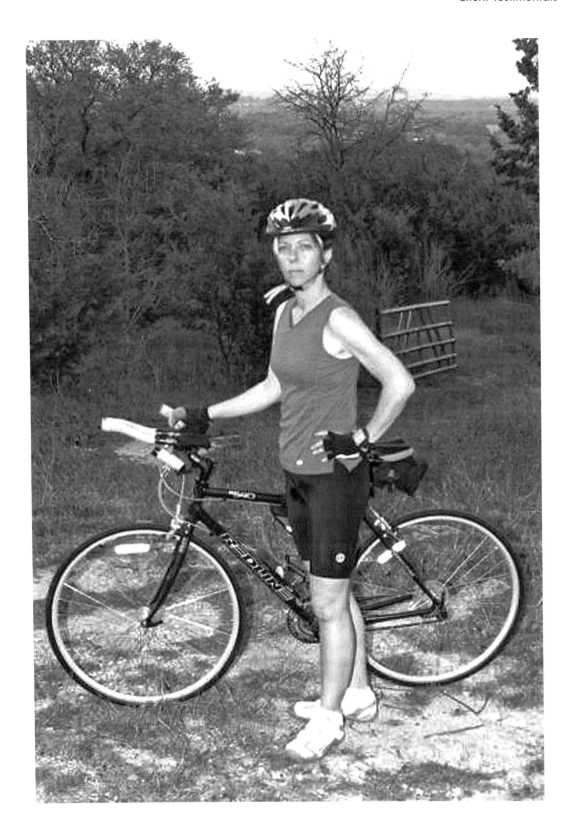

My excessive weight gain began in 1999. After contracting a skin infection, I was placed on a high dose of corticosteroids for several months. Prior to taking steroids, I had a healthy height-weight ratio of 5' 7" and 145 lb; however, while taking steroids I quickly gained 45 lb. This weight gain combined with my illness led to a more sedentary lifestyle, which in turn led to eating a typical American diet of fast food and fried food. As I gained more weight, this cluster of events began a vicious cycle. Over the next two years my weight spiraled out of control, my highest weight reaching 242 lb (body mass index, 37.9). This weight was recorded by my doctor, who ironically was treating me for back and foot pain. These conditions were a direct result of my morbid obesity.

I continued my attempts at exercise and diet for the next four years. During this time I went to a behavior clinic, was prescribed diet pills, consistently exercised at the gym, and even completed a Weight Watchers program. Each of these produced some degree of success, followed by immediate regression.

By the end of a six-year period, I had trigger-point pain requiring injections in my back, plantar fasciitis, metabolic syndrome, high blood pressure and cholesterol, advanced endometrial hyperplasia, fibroid tumors, dysmenorrhea, anemia, and renal insufficiency (as a result of renal toxicity from taking cholesterol medication). My kidneys were no longer able to tolerate cholesterol medication, and after I stopped taking cholesterol medication, my triglycerides rose to 527. My cholesterol ratio could no longer be measured because my triglycerides became so elevated. My blood glucose was 98, indicating borderline diabetes.

With the support of my physicians and sister, I made the decision to have Roux-en-Y gastric bypass. Due to postoperative complications, I spent five days in the hospital rather than the two-day norm. As for most patients, my exercise program began while I was in the hospital with the famous "hallway walks." When I was discharged, I was told that activity equals exercise, so my initial exercise program was measured by laps around the driveway, minutes on the treadmill, use of an elliptical trainer and recumbent bike, and performance of general household activities.

During the first four postoperative weeks I felt lousy: My body was adjusting to the rapid weight loss and nutritional changes. During the first two weeks after surgery, I lost 22 lb and no longer required any medications and my back and foot pain abated. Over the next few months I continued to lose approximately 1 lb per day.

For the first three months following surgery, I continued my exercise program at home using my elliptical trainer, recumbent bike, and weight set. I continued to gain strength and endurance but was having difficulty gaining abdominal strength. This weakness prompted me to schedule a personal training session with Megan Thiedeman, an exercise physiologist. This was a decision that proved to have a profound impact on the rest of my life. I was very nervous during my first session with Megan; however, she was very patient with me and taught me many exercises that I could perform at home.

I continued these exercises for two weeks, along with the exercise program I had previously been following. I then fell off the exercise "wagon" and did not do any form of exercise for two weeks. I noticed that my weight loss completely ceased when I stopped exercising. At this point, I had already lost 70 lb and was only 20 lb from reaching my personal weight goal. This plateau in my weight loss helped me recognize, without a doubt, that exercise was a "must" if I wanted to reach and maintain my weight goal.

My next step was to immediately join a gym. Signing up for a one-year membership, I made a commitment to myself that I would follow the exercise program set for me at least five days a week. As part of my program, I scheduled occasional personal training sessions with Megan in order to continue to upgrade my program. With this consistent exercise program, my energy level began to soar and my strength continued to increase. I included metabolic testing, both a resting metabolic rate and VO2 fitness testing, as part of my training protocol. This allowed my trainer to design an appropriate exercise program that would continue to assist me with my weight-loss efforts. I found these tests to be a valuable tool in helping me learn how many calories my body actually needed and how many calories I was burning each day in my normal activities. These tests also helped me to recognize how to exercise more efficiently, to ensure I wasn't overtraining, and to apply appropriate nutritional guidelines for continued weight loss and achieving my fitness goals.

When I joined the gym, my weight was 160 lb. I was only able to walk on the treadmill and use an elliptical trainer for about 15 minutes. My goal was to be able to run again. I set a personal goal to begin running when I weighed 150 lb. Once I reached 150 lb, I was still too self-conscious to attempt jogging on the treadmill in the gym where everyone could see me, so off to the track I went one Saturday morning. I was elated when I saw that I could actually move my body in a forward-running motion. I went back to the gym the following Monday with the mindset "if I can jog around the track, what else can I accomplish?" I gained the confidence I needed to be able to run in front of others and never looked back.

My trainer, Megan, continued to motivate me and I learned new things with each training session. I also learned by watching her train others and would incorporate some of those exercises into my own program. My first goal was to complete a 5K race (3.1-mile running race). This would be my first competitive event since high school, nearly 20 years ago. Megan gave me the committed guidance and coaching I needed to achieve this goal.

As I continued to follow my program, I was able to reach my personal goal weight eight months after my gastric bypass surgery. I had lost a total of 102 lb and was now completely hooked on exercise. My morning workouts were no longer enough. With the longer summer days having arrived, I enjoyed the addition of an evening bike ride or swim. Megan had mentioned that she was training for a triathlon. I thought to myself, "If she can complete one, what's stopping me?" After all, I was already running, cycling, and swimming. I then turned my focus toward completing a very short triathlon.

I completed my 5K and short triathlon just nine months after my surgery. I found that my energy level continued to increase with each exercise session I completed. Reaching my weight-loss goal and being able to compete in athletic events gave me a sense of achievement and a belief that that I could accomplish anything. Since my surgery I have now completed a half-marathon, the Hotter than Hell bike ride (60 miles), and a full marathon. With each event I complete, my personal confidence continues to grow. This degree of confidence influences all areas of my life.

To guide me in my training for my first half marathon, I joined a training program offered by one of the local sporting goods stores. I found it inspiring to be able to run with a group in which nobody knew me as a gastric bypass patient. Through the training for all of my sporting events, I have continued to receive valuable guidance and coaching from my trainers and extended support from my training partners. I have found that having the ongoing support of fitness-minded people is a key component in maintaining my motivation to exercise.

Completing the half marathon was of significant importance to me, since I achieved it one year and 10 days after my initial consultation with my gastric bypass surgeon. I told him that my completion of this event was my "anniversary gift" to him. I am committed to completing an athletic event to celebrate this date annually for as long as my body will allow.

Balancing my nutrition has been my greatest obstacle during my intense training periods for these events. I received enormous amounts of conflicting information from many of the medical professionals contributing to my care. My surgeon and dietician at the surgeon's office recommended a high-protein, low-carb diet, while my nephrologist who was treating my kidney stones recommended a high-carb, low-protein diet. The dietician affiliated with the training group recommended a formula for incorporating more carbs into my diet on the basis of the distances I was running. All of the information given to me by these professionals was very confusing. Following the diet set forth by my surgeon left me feeling depleted. On one of my afternoon bike rides I reached a point at which, after riding my bike only 1 mile, I no longer had enough energy to power my muscles to keep riding. Once again, I sought advice from my trainer, Megan, and she was able to help me balance all of the advice from the health professionals with the demands that were being placed on my body by my intense physical training. I also learned the hard lesson of not overtraining. Once my diet and exercise program were properly balanced, my energy level and athletic abilities began to climb once again.

I have been told by the trainers and my surgeon that the exercise and training program I began following weight-loss surgery is not typical for most patients. My experience has been that it *is* typical for *me*, fitting my personality and what I had envisioned for myself prior to my surgery. When I was morbidly obese, I could not believe that those words were used to describe me and could not believe that I was actually a candidate for gastric bypass surgery. Because I had been an athlete throughout my high school years and had ridden my bike consistently throughout my years in college, I was shocked that this had happened to me. When I would see a picture of myself, I could not believe it was me, as I had never felt like the fat person that other people saw. I had always avoided mirrors at all costs. The mirrors in the gym are more bearable now, and they help me stay focused on remaining optimally fit and healthy through regular exercise and proper nutrition. I knew prior to my surgery that I would need to exercise in order to get my body back into the shape that I envisioned. Many people will never train for a competitive event; however, my belief is that each person should evaluate why they are contemplating weight-loss surgery and recognize that regular exercise after surgery will improve their ability to reach their ultimate goal.

Many people use the excuse of not having enough time to exercise. I made a commitment to go to the gym each morning as the first priority in my day. Completing my exercise program and being around others who are enthusiastic about exercise increases my energy level and mental capacity throughout the day. However, I am no different than the next person: I have encountered physical, emotional, and financial stresses during the course of my fitness journey. In addition, like most people, my time is limited, but I have found that attaining my physical and emotional well-being through exercise makes everything else fall into place.

The training for and completion of sporting events has been a tremendous healing emotional journey. Each week of my training continues to be a journey. While I complete the training protocol for each event, I have plenty of time during my runs, bike rides, and swims to mentally process and reflect on where I have come from and where I am going. Through this process I have come to the realization that although I like and appreciate the support of others through this lifelong journey, it truly is an individual battle, fought by one person—me. I am the only person that is responsible for what happens to me. I will continue with the commitment I have made to myself.

After in-depth consideration, I made the decision to allow my surgeon to cut me open, amputate my stomach and rearrange my upper gastrointestinal tract. Going into surgery, I knew the risks involved and that I would permanently change my life. This is what I wanted. I also knew that there were many foods that I once enjoyed eating that I would not be able to eat again for the rest of my life. I also accepted the fact that in my future there may be some additional medical challenges that I will have to endure as a result of having weight-loss surgery. This was a big decision that was a long time in the making. Through my exercise program, I have been met with the preconceived notion by both fitness staff and gym members that surgical weight-loss patients have it "easier" than the medical weight-loss patients. As a previous medical weight-loss patient and now a surgical weight-loss patient, I can say with assurance that the challenges faced as a surgical weight-loss patient are significant. Not to undermine the work that the medical weight-loss patients put into their programs, but as a surgical weight-loss patient I, too, have had to put a high degree of work into my program. Although the numbers on the scale may change more quickly following surgery, the challenge and process of losing weight and maintaining weight loss is not easier; it is just different. I had no insurance or other financial support in this endeavor.

Other than my sister, I had no family support for my decision to have weight-loss surgery. The total commitment to go through this process came from me, and I carried this commitment over to my exercise program. With no insurance to "fund" my surgery, I use my exercise program as "insurance" that my surgery will have a successful outcome. During my own personal journey, the best support I found was within the walls of the gym. The ongoing support I receive from my trainers and other gym members is one of the ultimate factors in keeping me motivated.

I continue to feel compelled to compete, as I have a personal commitment to strive for excellence in everything that I do. As long as I am physically able to compete, there will always be a race to train for and a new personal goal to meet. Competing against other athletes, especially those who do not know that I carry the label "formerly morbid obese gastric bypass patient" gives me a sense of accomplishment that I would have never believed was possible for myself.

Routine, consistent exercise has played a valuable role in my weight-loss success. Exercise will always be the key to preventing my regaining weight, which is one of my biggest fears. My life has changed to one of full activity, rather than just merely existing. Following this program has helped me achieve a normal height/weight ratio of 5' 7" and 130 lb (20.4 body mass index), with 14 percent body fat. I feel terrific, and I love my new life. I plan to participate in many more fitness events that will help me continue to give meaning to my workouts. I surround myself with people who love exercise as much as I do and who support me in my efforts and goals. In our sedentary society, this is not an easy thing to do, but I must keep moving forward. In closing, I encourage everyone who reads this to get moving!

STEFANIE ALVHEIM

I was sick of my sick way of eating and living. Even the exercise I was doing wasn't making a dent. After putting on numerous pounds I knew I had to do something about my weight as well as my health. As a mother I felt it necessary to lead by example, so I started a weight-loss program through a medically supervised weight-loss clinic. A good friend of mine who had also gained some weight during and even after her pregnancies was in the same boat. Together we were ready to try something new and make a change; this is when we started down the path of fitness together.

We both embraced the clinic's comprehensive approach to losing weight and being healthy. The clinic had providers of expertise on diet, exercise, and medical information (physicians) all under one roof, and each provider worked together to ensure our goals were being met. My friend and I availed ourselves of weekly support from each provider at the clinic, and it made a huge difference for us. The fitness professionals provided information tailored to our own issues and bodies and educated us about the most efficient ways each of us could eat better and burn calories and fat through exercise. We soon realized that we had been doing a lot of things wrong in our past approaches to weight loss.

Early in the process, I began working out with Julia Karlstad and she soon became my main touchstone. Julia was able to track my progress every week and make adjustments accordingly. Having such a dedicated and professional trainer motivated me to work out regularly. I was never bored and was constantly amazed by Julia's repertoire of exercises. She rarely had me do the same thing twice! I convinced my friend to join me in my workouts with Julia. It didn't take long before my friend to experienced positive results. We were able to dramatically improve our muscle tone as well as our core strength. I became more confident about my ability to perform complex exercises. I also loved the tandem workouts with my friend and found myself pushing harder because I had a partner. Julia's enthusiasm for fitness was infectious.

It's been well over a year into this adventure, and I can attest that working with a partner/friend has been a huge plus in maintaining a constant, routine exercise regimen and motivating me to lose weight, eat healthier, and become a physically strong woman! My friend and I joke that we can't even say that our relationships with our husbands have given us so much. Being friends and a workout partners has been a tremendous blessing—we both relentlessly support and motivate one another! I personally had no idea how my life would change when, that fortuitous day at the gym, I mentioned that I was going to try to make a change and visit a weight-loss clinic. Little did I know that a year and a half later, I would still be walking side-by-side with my friend on the treadmill and each of us would be 40+ pounds lighter. Working out with a partner (it has to be someone you like) has made all the difference for me. I have another layer of accountability, but it's packaged as a loving, fun friend.

Client Testimonials

MEG LESIEUR

I have always considered myself overweight. Growing up, I was fairly active through high school. I mainly rode my bike everywhere and kept my weight around 145 lb. It wasn't until the birth of my first child that I started to gain weight and keep it on. Giving birth to my second child before I worked off the weight I had gained from my first pregnancy compounded the problem. My weight continued to fluctuate for the next 20 years. I would try one diet or another and sometimes accomplish significant weight loss, only to regain what I had lost, plus more weight.

During this time I would mix in some type of exercise, usually walking, while dieting. About five and a half years ago (2003), I started focusing on eating healthy and trying to lose weight, but it didn't matter what I did. I couldn't lose more than 20 lb. At this time I was so obese that any type of physical activity exhausted me. That's when I seriously started looking at weight-loss surgery. By the time I finished my research, visited the doctor, had all the tests done, etc., I was able to get on a waiting list in the summer of 2005. On June 6, 2006, I had laparoscopic Roux-en-Y gastric bypass surgery. I actually was 356 lb when I was weighed at the doctor's office around April 2006. I'm sure I weighed more than that at some point, but my scale at home only went up to 350 lb. The day of my surgery, I weighed 336 lb.

Fortunately, I didn't have any complications following the surgery. I was in the hospital for three days. In the days following the surgery, I did everything the doctor told me to: I walked and drank the appropriate amount of liquids and I slowly added soft foods. I started to see the scale going down, which was an exhilarating feeling. In the first part of July (one month after my surgery) I went to an Obesity Help conference in San Antonio. There were presentations from many different experts in the field of bariatrics. It was at this conference that I ran across Julia Karlstad. She presented a lecture explaining how exercise was the key component to long-term weight loss. I decided to meet with Julia at a medical clinic where she worked, and I signed up to undergo the metabolic tests they offered. These tests allowed me to see where I was physically as well as how my metabolism was working. I found out my resting metabolic rate was way below normal, about 1,300 calories. No wonder I was having so much trouble losing weight! Even if I were to follow a 1,200 calorie a day diet, I would have no real chance of losing any significant weight. Especially seeing that 3,500 calories make up one pound of fat.

Rx Fitness for Weight Loss: The Medically Sound Solution to Get Fit and Save Your Life

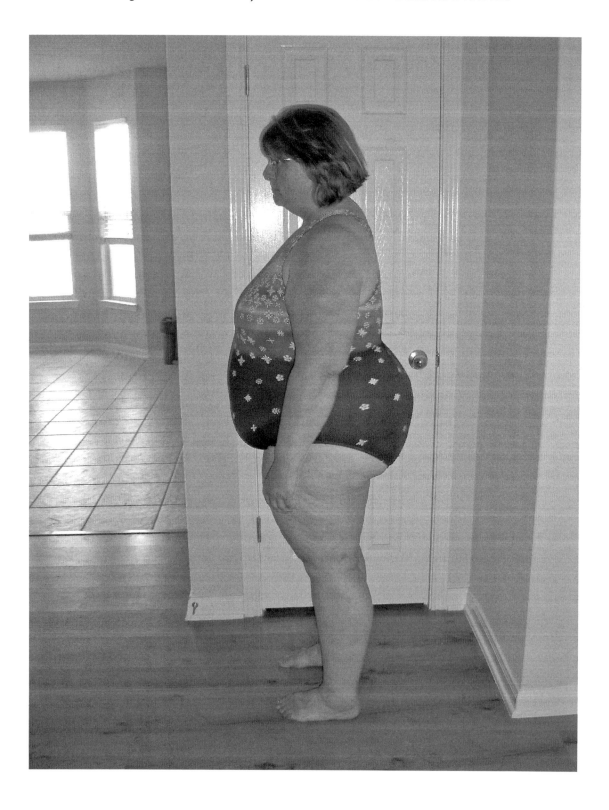

Client Testimonials

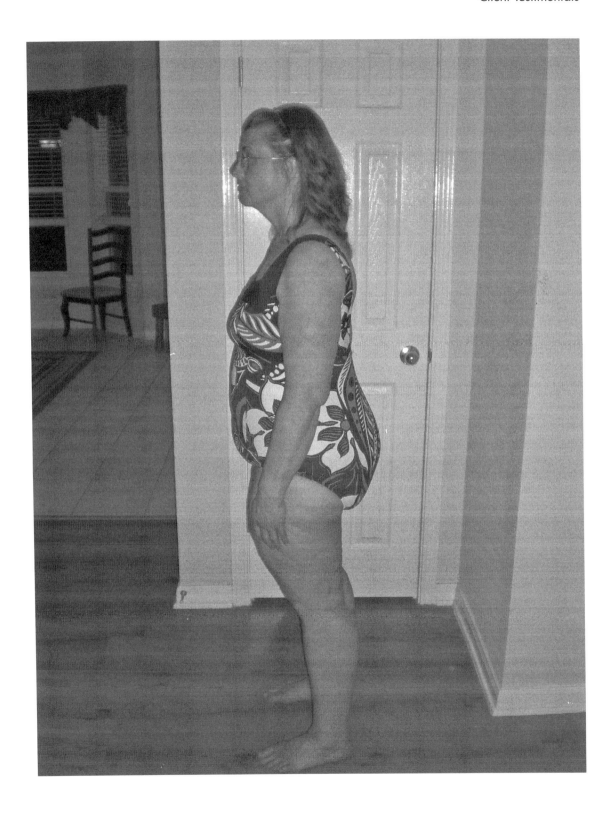

Julia recommended I start a weight-training program to build some lean muscle, which would ultimately help increase my metabolism. Weight training had always intimidated me because I didn't know what to do or how to do it; however, Julia walked me through every exercise to make sure I was comfortable with each one. She didn't think any question was silly, and she really made me feel like I could do this exercise "thing"! Having a personal trainer has given me the confidence and belief that my weight-loss efforts and exercise program will really work this time. Julia has encouraged me every step of the way and is always enthusiastic about my progress. When I re-tested my metabolic rates nine months later, my resting rate had actually increased to over 1,700!

Julia, along with the other providers at this weight-loss clinic, were instrumental in both preparing me for life after surgery—what to expect and the steps I needed to take in order to keep the weight off for good! Julia stressed the importance of keeping up a physical training program. I've maintained a rigorous physical training program to facilitate my recovery. I go to the gym every work day before work, alternating cardio workouts with the weight-training routine Julia designed for me. I get a new routine every 6-8 weeks to keep my body from "getting in a rut." My eating has not been perfect; I still need to work on that, but without the exercise I would not have lost over 170 lb. I feel better when I exercise and I am definitely looking better too!

Appendix A
Recommendations for Workout Apparel, Accessories, and Equipment

These are strictly my own personal recommendations. I offer them without any obligation to any other person or company. I have personally purchased and used the brands I recommend and have had good experiences with them, but there are, of course, no guarantees. You, the reader, ultimately need to make your own personal judgments about what equipment, clothing, accessories, or other items are best for you.

Workout Apparel
- *Fitness Clothing*

Under Armour (www.underarmour.com)
Nike (www.nike.com)

- *Running Shoes*

Saucony
Mizuno
Asics
Brooks

- *Walking Shoes*

New Balance
Saucony
Accessories

- *Heart Rate Monitor*

Polar Heart Rate Monitor, Model FS2 (www.polar-heartrate-monitors.com)

- *Sunglasses*

Smith (www.smithoptics.com)
Nike (www.nike.com)

- *iPod*

Apple iPod Shuffle (www.apple.com/ipodshuffle/)

- *GPS "All in One" Watch*

Garmin Model Forerunner 305 (www.garmin.com)
Equipment

- *Treadmill, Elliptical, or Stationary Bike*

TRUE (www.truefitness.com)
BLADEZ (www.ebladez.com)
Life Fitness (www.lifefitness.com)
NordicTrack (www.nordictrack.com)
PRECORE (www.precore.com)

- *Mountain Bike*

Trek
Raleigh

- *Racing Bike*

Schwinn
Cannondale
Trek

- *Bike Odometer or Computer*

CATEYE (www.cateye.com)

- *Total Gym*

Cable-driven with plate-loaded machine (dual adjustable cable by Life Fitness, PRECORE, or Free Motion)

- *Place to Purchase Home or Functional Fitness Equipment*

Power-Systems (www.power-systems.com)

Appendix B
Rate of Perceived Exertion (RPE): How Hard You Feel You Are Exercising

0	**Rest:** No exertion at all
1	**Very light:** Can converse with little or no effort
2	**Light:** Can converse with very little effort
3	**Moderate:** Conversation requires some effort
4	**Somewhat hard:** Conversation requires effort but still able to carry on a conversation without being winded
5	**Hard:** Conversation requires quite a bit of effort
6	**Harder:** Conversation requires quite a bit of effort
7	**Very hard:** Conversation requires a lot of effort
8	**Very hard:** Conversation requires a lot of effort
9	**Very hard:** Conversation very difficult; nearly unable to talk
10	**Very, very hard:** maximal effort required and unable to talk

Glossary

A1c test   Also known as *hemoglobin A1C* or *HbA1C*, this test evaluates the average amount of glucose in the blood over the last two to three months by measuring the concentration of glycosylated hemoglobin. As glucose circulates in the blood, some of it spontaneously binds to hemoglobin A (the primary form of hemoglobin in adults).

Aerobic exercise   Activity that requires moving large muscle groups in a rhythmic motion for an extended period of time; involving, utilizing, or increasing oxygen consumption for metabolic processes in the human body.

acromion   An anatomical feature of the scapula; also called the *acromial process*. The acromion forms the summit of the shoulder and is a large, somewhat triangular or oblong process.

activities of daily living (ADLs)   Movements or actions performed on a daily basis; e.g., getting out of bed, climbing stairs, cooking, taking a shower, walking.

anaerobic exercise   Exercise at high intensity during which the need of muscle metabolism for oxygen exceeds the capacity of the circulation to supply it and thus an oxygen debt is incurred.

anaerobic threshold   High level of exercise at which lactic acid begins to build up in the blood; this happens when lactic acid is produced faster than it can be metabolized.

anterior pelvic tilt   Exaggerated inward curve of the spine in the low back or lumbar area, typically the result of muscle imbalances and very common in overweight individuals due to their excess weight.

arm ergometer   A piece of exercise equipment designed to meet the needs of individuals who aren't able to use their lower body for exercise, offering a cardio workout using the upper body instead of the legs. Essentially designed as a "bike" for the arms; most arm ergometers offer wheelchair access. See also *upper extremity bike*.

arrhythmias   Any group of conditions in which the electrical activity of the heart is irregular or is faster or slower than normal. Some arrhythmias are life-threatening medical emergencies that can cause cardiac arrest and sudden death. Others cause aggravating symptoms, such as an awareness of a different heart beat, or palpitations, which can be annoying. Some are quite minor and are regarded as benign.

arthritis   Joint inflammation causing pain and swelling.

athlete   A person trained or skilled in exercises, sports, or games requiring physical strength, agility, or stamina.

ballistic movement   Jerky, bouncing movement.

bariatric chair   A chair especially designed for an obese individual; this chair is wider than the normal chair and sturdy enough to withstand excess body weight.

bariatrics   A field of medicine that deals with the causes, prevention, and treatment of obesity.

bariatric surgery   Also known as *weight-loss surgery*, this term refers to various surgical procedures performed to treat obesity. For individuals who have not been unable to achieve significant weight loss through diet modifications and exercise programs alone, bariatric surgery may help an individual attain a more healthy body weight. There are a number of surgical options available to treat obesity, each with their advantages and pitfalls. In general, bariatric surgery is successful in producing weight loss (often substantial), although one must consider operative risk (including mortality) and side effects before making the decision to pursue this treatment option. Usually, bariatric surgical procedures can be carried out safely.

beta blocker   Any of various substances that interfere with the action of the beta receptors; used primarily to reduce the heart rate for the prevention, management, and/or treatment of angina, hypertension, or arrhythmias. This medication is also used, on occasion, to manage migraine headaches.

bioelectrical impedance   A form of body composition testing in which an electrical current is passed through the body. The more muscle a person has, the more water that can be held, thus the faster the current will travel through the body. The more fat on a person's body, the more resistance to the current. The impedance determines one's body fat, lean muscle mass, and water weight.

blood glucose   The concentration of glucose (sugar) in the blood, measured in milligrams (mg) of glucose per 100 milliliters (mL) of blood.

blood pressure   The pressure exerted by the blood against the walls of the blood vessels; measured in millimeters of mercury (mm Hg).

- **diastolic blood pressure**   Ventricular relaxation of the heart; as it relates to blood pressure, it is the bottom number/value in a blood pressure reading.
- **systolic blood pressure**   Ventricular contraction of the ventricles; as it relates to blood pressure, it is the top number/value in a blood pressure reading.

body bars   Weighted bar-like piece of strength equipment; often covered with foam padding.

body composition   The percentages of fat, bone, and muscle in a human body. The percentage of fat, body fat percentage, is of most interest because it can be very helpful in judging an individual's health as well as excess body weight.

body mass index (BMI)   A measurement that is the ratio of the weight of the body in kilograms (kg) to the square of its height in meters (m^2). Often used to determine weight classification (e.g., underweight, normal weight, overweight, obese). Originally developed by the Metropolitan Life Insurance Company in 1959 for creation of a height/weight table.

body weight   The relative heaviness of one's body, generally measured in kilograms (kg) or pounds (lb).

brachial artery   The main artery of the upper arm; a continuation of the axillary artery, it branches into the radial and ulnar arteries at the elbow.

bulging disc   A spinal disorder characterized by an intervertebral disc bulging out from the vertebrae.

bursitis   Inflammation of the bursa (a bodily pouch or sac between a tendon and a bone).

calipers   An instrument for measuring the thickness or depth of skin folds; one can determine body fat through the use of calipers. In this method of body fat testing the skin is pinched in predetermined locations on the body (three spots or seven spots), and then an equation is used to determine the percentage of total body fat.

callisthenic   Light exercises designed to promote general fitness.

cancer   Any of various malignant neoplasms characterized by the increase of anaplastic cells, which tend to invade surrounding tissue and metastasize to new body sites.

carotid artery   Either of the two large arteries, one on each side of the head, that carry blood to the head and that divide into an external branch supplying the neck, face, and other external parts, and an internal branch supplying the brain, eye, and other internal parts.

cardio   Of, relating to, or involving the heart and blood vessels. Also, exercises used, designed, or performed to cause a temporary increase in heart rate (a cardiovascular workout).

cardiology   The medical study of the structure, function, and disorders of the heart.

cervical disc disease   Disease of the cervical spine, related to the neck.

cholesterol   A white crystalline substance, $C_{27}H_{45}OH$, found in animal tissues and various foods, that is normally synthesized by the liver and is important as a constituent of cell membranes and a precursor to steroid hormones. Its level in the bloodstream can influence the pathogenesis of certain conditions, such as the development of atherosclerotic plaque and coronary artery disease.

- **HDL**   High-density lipoproteins; the "good" cholesterol. A high level of HDL in the blood is thought to lower the risk of coronary artery disease.
- **LDL**   Low-density lipoproteins; the "bad" cholesterol. A high level in the blood is thought to be related to various pathogenic conditions.
- **VLDL**   Very low-density lipoproteins; "bad" cholesterol. VLDL contains the highest level of triglycerides.

cholesterol ratios   The total cholesterol/HDL and LDL/HDL ratios, which are very helpful in determining the overall risk of developing atherosclerosis.

co-morbidity   The presence of one or more disorders (or diseases) in addition to a primary disease or disorder.

comprehensive metabolic panel (CMP)   A standard panel of 14 blood tests that serves as an initial broad screening tool for physicians. Because a CMP is often ordered as a routine part of an annual physical examination or checkup, over time the CMP provides an important baseline of a patient's physiological status. Any changes or abnormal results—in particular combinations of abnormal results—provides important initial data for differential diagnosis, in which case more specialized tests may be indicated. In and of itself, however, a CMP provides important, albeit general, information on the status of an individual's kidney function, liver function, and electrolyte and fluid balance.

compression sleeve   An elasticized sleeve customized to fit a particular body part; often used on the arm to prevent and/or treat lymphedema.

concentric motion   A movement that contracts, or shortens, a muscle or group of muscles.

contracture   A condition of fixed high resistance to passive stretching of a muscle, resulting from fibrosis of the tissues supporting the muscles or joints or from disorders of muscle fiber; also, an abnormal, often permanent shortening of the tissues, as occurs as a result of scar tissue, that results in distortion or deformity.

contraindicated movement   Physical activity that is inadvisable; a contraindicated movement may cause more harm to the particular affected area of the body or worsen a medical condition.

core muscles   Abdominal, back, and pelvis muscles make up the core; strong core muscles make it easier to do most physical activities.

degenerative disc disease (DDD)   Degeneration of an intervertebral disc; also referred to as *degenerative disc disease (DDD) of the spine.* DDD is a common disorder of the lower spine, and in some people, can cause low back pain and/or leg pain (sciatica). Disc degeneration can also lead to disorders such as lumbar or cervical spinal stenosis (narrowing of the spinal canal that houses the spinal cord and nerve roots; spondylolisthesis (forward slippage of the disc and vertebra); retrolisthesis (backward slippage of the disc and vertebra); and osteoarthritis, in which bone spurs grow adjacent to the discs and pinch or put pressure on the nearby nerve roots or spinal canal.

diabetes mellitus   A variable disorder of carbohydrate metabolism caused by a combination of hereditary and environmental factors and usually characterized by inadequate secretion or utilization of insulin, by excessive urine production, by excessive amounts of sugar in the blood and urine, and by thirst, hunger, and loss of weight.

- **gestational diabetes**   Glucose intolerance during pregnancy; a form of diabetes that affects pregnant women who have never had diabetes before. There is no known specific cause, but it's believed that the hormones produced during pregnancy reduce a woman's receptivity to insulin, resulting in high blood glucose (sugar).
- **type I**   Usually diagnosed in childhood. The body makes little or no insulin, and daily injections of insulin are needed to sustain life.
- **type II**   Far more common than type I, which usually occurs in adulthood. The pancreas does not make enough insulin to keep blood glucose levels normal, often because the body does not respond well to the insulin. Many people with type II diabetes do not know they have it, although it is a serious condition.

dislocation   The act of displacing a bone from its normal position.

dorsiflex   The act of bending a joint, especially a joint between the bones of a limb, so that the angle between them is decreased.

dorsiflexion   Flexion or bending toward the extensor aspect of a limb, as on the hand or foot.

drop foot   A deficit in turning the ankle and toes upward (dorsiflexion); also called *foot drop*. Conditions that may lead to foot drop may be neurological, muscular, or anatomical in origin, often with significant overlap.

dual adjustable pulley system   A cable weight machine driven by a pulley system and designed to produce resistance from bilateral sides.

duodenal switch   Also known as *biliopancreatic diversion with duodenal switch* or the *DS procedure*, the duodenal switch is a weight-loss surgery that alters the gastrointestinal tract with two approaches: a restrictive aspect and a malabsorptive aspect. The restrictive portion of the surgery reduces the stomach along the greater curvature so that the volume is approximately one-third to one-fifth of the original capacity. The malabsorptive portion of the surgery reroutes a lengthy portion of the small intestine, creating two separate pathways and one common pathway. The shorter of the two pathways, the digestive loop, takes food from the stomach to the large intestine. The much longer pathway, the biliopancreatic loop, carries bile from the liver to the common path. The common path, or common channel, is a stretch of small intestine usually 75-150 centimeters (cm) long in which the contents of the digestive path mix with the bile from the biliopancreatic loop before emptying into the large intestine. The objective of this arrangement is to reduce the amount of time the body has to capture calories from food in the small intestine and to selectively limit the absorption of fat.

eccentric motion   An action that lengthens or elongates the muscle; occurs when the muscle is resisting gravity.

environment   The conditions, influences, and things that surround; all other external factors that affect an organism at a given time; the social and cultural conditions that shape the life of a person or population.

fitness assessment   An evaluation that measures one's physical state.

- **balance**   Assesses physical equilibrium; the ability to retain one's balance.
- **flexibility**   Assesses the physical ability to move a joint through its full range of motion.
- **posture**   Assesses the position one hold's the body while standing in an upright right position.
- **strength**   Assesses one's ability to produce force with muscles upon a given object.
- **VO2 max**   Assesses one's ability to uptake a maximal amount of oxygen during a cardiovascular fitness assessment; the more oxygen the body can uptake and utilize, the better the individual's cardiovascular condition ("heart health").

flexibility   The ability to move a joint through a full range of motion.

flexion   The act of a muscle or muscle group bending a joint or limb in the body and decreasing the angle at a joint.

fracture   A break in a bone.

frozen shoulder   Inflammation between the joint capsule and the peripheral articular shoulder cartilage; causes pain whether in motion or at rest. Also called *adhesive capsulitis*.

gastric bypass   A surgical procedure used for treatment of morbid obesity, consisting of the severance of the upper stomach, attachment of the small upper pouch of the stomach to the jejunum, and closure of the distal part of the stomach.

gastric sleeve   A surgical weight-loss procedure in which the stomach is reduced to about 35 percent of its original size by surgical removal of a large portion of the stomach, following the major curve of the stomach. The open edges of new stomach are then attached (often with surgical staples) to form a banana-shaped sleeve or tube. The procedure permanently reduces the size of the stomach.

geriatrics   The branch of medicine that deals with the diagnosis and treatment of diseases and problems specific to the aged.

girth measurements   The measurement around anything. As it relates to health and fitness, the measurement around certain body parts (i.e. waist, hips, thighs, arms, chest, or neck)

glucometer   A device for determining the approximate concentration of glucose (sugar) in the blood. It is a key element of home blood-glucose monitoring by people with diabetes mellitus or with proneness to hypoglycemia. A small drop of blood obtained by pricking the skin with a lancet is placed on a disposable test strip, which the glucometer reads and uses to calculate the blood glucose level.

glutes   The buttocks muscles.

glycemic index   A system that ranks foods by the speed at which their carbohydrates are converted into glucose in the body; a measure of the effects of foods on blood glucose levels. The higher the food falls on the glycemic index, the more rapidly the conversion of carbohydrate in the body, which initially causes a spike in the blood glucose level.

goniometer   An instrument for measuring angles. As it relates to health and fitness it is generally used to measure the angle between two joints thus helping assess one's flexibility or range of motion in a particular joint.

Gulick measuring tape   Device that makes it easy for anyone to accurately measure various body dimensions. It eliminates the guesswork by applying a constant tension to the measuring tape. When used properly, accurate measurements are possible no matter who is doing the measuring.

hamstrings   The two tendons behind each knee and their associated muscles (biceps femoris, semitendinosus, and semimembranosus).

heart disease   A structural or functional abnormality of the heart, or of the blood vessels supplying the heart, that impairs its normal functioning.

heart rate   The number of heart beats in a period of time; generally measured in, and referred to as, beats per minute (bpm).

- **ambient**   One-minute heart rate in a seated and resting position.
- **maximum**   The highest heart rate one can get during maximal physical exertion or the highest number of times the heart can beat in 1 minute. One's maximum heart rate is believed to decrease with age; 220 minus age (220 – age) is a classic equation that can be used to calculate your estimated maximum heart rate. The maximum heart rate can also be used to calculate the target heart rate.
- **recovery**   The heart rate your body will return to after exercise; usually taken 2 minutes after exercise. For example, if your exercising heart rate is 154 bpm and then you stop exercising for 2 minutes and your heart rate decreased after the 2 minutes to 105 bpm, 105 bpm would be your recovery heart rate.
- **resting**   One-minute heart rate in a resting position; usually taken first thing in the morning right after one wakes up and before getting out of bed.
- **target**   The heart rate calculated from one's maximal heart rate determined through metabolic VO2 testing. This is the rate that produces cardiovascular benefits; in other words, the heart and lungs will benefit when exercising at this level. One's fit zone is based on the target heart rate. Depending on the individual's fitness level, 50-85 percent of maximum heart rate is used to

calculate the target heart rate. Thus, you can calculate target heart rate using the max heart rate or Karvonen method equations.

heart rate monitor   A monitoring device that allows tracking of the heart rate in real time. The monitor generally consists of a chest strap and a watch. There is a transmitter in the chest strap, and the receiver in the watch displays the heart rate.

hernia   The protrusion of an organ or tissue through an opening in its surrounding walls, occurs most frequently in the abdominal region.

herniated disc   A tear in the outer, fibrous ring (annulus fibrosus) of an intervertebral disc, allowing the soft, central portion (nucleus pulposus) to bulge out; also referred to as *slipped disc*.

hip flexors   A group of muscles that act to flex the femur, the long bone in the thigh that connects the pelvis and knee. They act to pull the knee upward.

hip replacement   A surgical procedure in which the hip joint is replaced by a prosthetic implant; this surgery is generally performed to relieve arthritis pain or fix severe joint damage.

Hiss-Compress exercises   A method of exercise recommended for pregnant women, also known as *C-Curve*; helps relieve discomfort during pregnancy and prepare for labor.

hydrostatic weighing   A method of measuring body composition in which an individual is weighed under water. Since the density of fat is lighter than the density of water and the density of lean tissue is heavier than water, one's body composition can be determined through this method of testing.

hypertension   Arterial disease in which chronic high blood pressure is the primary symptom.

hypertrophic cardiomyopathy (HCM)   A disease of the myocardium (the muscle of the heart) in which a portion of the myocardium is hypertrophied (thickened) without any obvious cause. Although perhaps most famous as a leading cause of sudden cardiac death in athletes, HCM's more important significance is that it is a cause of sudden unexpected cardiac death in all age groups as well as a cause of disabling cardiac symptoms.

hypoglycemia   An abnormally low level of glucose in the blood.

hypothyroidism A disease state caused by insufficient production of thyroid hormone by the thyroid gland.

impingement A very common pain in the shoulder resulting from pressure on the rotator cuff from part of the shoulder blade (scapula) as the arm is lifted.

indirect calorimetry A technique used to measure metabolic rates in which a gas analyzer measures oxygen consumption and the amount of carbon dioxide expired. The measurement of gas exchange determines energy expenditure both at rest and during exercise.

insulin A polypeptide hormone produced by the pancreas that regulates the metabolism of glucose and other nutrients.

interval training Bursts of high-intensity activity alternating with short periods of low- to moderate-intensity activity. This type of training is very effective in building cardiovascular fitness and increasing the body's fat-burning capacity and overall caloric burn.

Karvonen method A method of calculating one's target heart rate (THR) that factors in one's resting heart rate (HR_{rest}), theoretical max heart rate (HR_{max}), and the intensity level at which one intends to train. The Karvonen method calculation formula is: $THR = [(HR_{max} - HR_{rest}) \times \% \text{ Intensity}] + HR_{rest}$.

Kegel exercises Named after Dr. Arnold Kegel, these exercises are designed to strengthen the pelvic floor muscles in women and thus make birth easier, enhance sexual enjoyment, and help prevent incontinence; they consist of contracting and relaxing the muscles that form part of the pelvic floor.

knee replacement A commonly performed operation done to relieve pain and disability from osteoarthritis or rheumatoid arthritis of the knee; the former is more common.

kyphosis Curvature of the upper spine, which can be either the result of bad posture or a structural anomaly in the spine.

LAP-BAND A form of restrictive weight-loss surgery involving the placement of a gastric band around the stomach; designed for obese patients with a body mass index (BMI) of 40 or greater or a BMI between 35-40 who also have co-morbidities known to improve with weight loss. The gastric band is an inflatable silicone prosthetic device, which is placed around the top portion of the stomach via keyhole laparoscopic surgery.

lat pulldown   A strength-training exercise for the upper back, often performed on a strength machine; the person performing the exercise sits facing the machine and pulls the bar down to the chin, keeping the back upright.

lipid panel   A blood test that measures lipids (fats and fatty substances) used as a source of energy by your body. Lipids include cholesterol, triglycerides, high-density lipoprotein (HDL), and low-density lipoprotein (LDL).

lordosis   An abnormal forward or increased curvature in the lumbar spine commonly referred to as *swayback* or *saddleback*; causes of lordosis include obesity, weak core muscles, pregnancy, and tight back and/or hamstring muscles.

low-impact activities   Activities that cause little to no stress on the body or joints.

lumpectomy   A common surgical procedure designed to remove a discrete lump, usually a tumor (benign or malignant), from an affected woman's or man's breast.

lymphedema   Swelling produced by an accumulation of lymph fluid in the soft tissue; a possible complication for anyone who has undergone lumpectomy or mastectomy.

mastectomy   Surgical removal of one or both breasts.

metabolism   The sum of the physical and chemical processes in an organism by which its material substance is produced, maintained, and destroyed, and by which energy is made available.

metabolize   To subject to metabolism; to change by metabolism.

mitochondria   Spherical or elongated organelles in the cytoplasm of nearly all eukaryotic cells; mitochondria contain genetic material and a number of enzymes important for cell metabolism, including those responsible for the conversion of food to usable energy. Since mitochondria break down food to produce energy, they can be considered the body's power houses.

modality   See *mode*.

mode   A particular type or form of something, i.e., walking is a form or mode of cardio exercise.

multiple sclerosis (MS)   A chronic degenerative disease of the central nervous system in which gradual destruction of myelin occurs in patches throughout the brain or spinal cord or both, interfering with the nerve pathways and causing muscular weakness, loss of coordination, and speech and visual disturbances. MS occurs chiefly in young adults and is thought to be caused by a defect in the immune system that may be of genetic or viral origin.

muscular dystrophy (MD)   Any of a group of progressive muscle disorders caused by a defect in one or more genes that control muscle function; characterized by gradual irreversible wasting of skeletal muscle.

myocardial infarction (MI)   Death of a region of the myocardium caused by an interruption in the supply of blood to the heart, usually as a result of a closing or blockage of a coronary artery; also called *cardiac infarction*.

neuropathy   A functional disturbance or pathological change in the peripheral nervous system, sometimes limited to non-inflammatory lesions as opposed to those of neuritis. In diabetics, neuropathy often leads to a tingly or numbness in the lower limbs. Proper foot care is very important for individuals who have neuropathy.

neutral alignment   A standing position in which the feet are shoulder width apart and toes are pointed forward, the shoulders are back, the chest is out, and the chin parallel to the floor. Hips, knees, and ankles should all fall in alignment with one another. This position is considered to be good posture; it is also the proper position for performing physical activity and exercise.

obesity   An increase in body weight beyond the limitation of skeletal and physical requirements, as the result of excessive accumulation of body fat.

obesity classifications   *Obesity* can be defined in absolute or relative terms. In practical settings, obesity is typically evaluated in absolute terms by measuring body mass index (BMI) and classified into one of three categories (class I, II, or III).

- **class I**   Obesity classification if BMI = 30 to 34.9.
- **class II**   Obesity classification if BMI = 35 to 39.9.

- **class III** Obesity classification if BMI is more than 40 and/or body weight is more than 100 lb over the individual's ideal body weight; also called *morbid obesity*.

one-rep maximum The amount of weight or force an individual can produce through one repetition of an exercise, usually specific to a strength-training exercise. For example, if the maximum amount of weight a person can lift during a bench press is 50 lb, 50 lb is the individual's one-rep maximum for the bench press.

osteoarthritis A form of arthritis characterized by chronic degeneration of the cartilage of the joints.

osteopenia A decrease in bone-mineral density that can be a precursor condition to osteoporosis; however, not every person diagnosed with osteopenia will develop osteoporosis.

osteophytes Bone spurs. Bony projections that form along joints.

osteoporosis A disorder in which the bones become increasingly porous, brittle, and subject to fracture, owing to loss of calcium and other mineral components, sometimes resulting in pain, decreased height, and skeletal deformities. Osteoporosis is common in older persons, primarily postmenopausal women, but is also associated with long-term steroid therapy and certain endocrine disorders.

overtraining This occurs when a person is doing too much exercise or training; symptoms include elevated resting heart rate, fatigue, decreased immune system, irritability, lack of a desire to exercise, and painful muscles. Unless training for a competition, over 2 hours of exercise on any given day for consecutive days is generally going to push an individual into an overtrained state, which may result in injury.

pediatrics The branch of medicine concerned with the development, care, and diseases of babies and children.

pelvic girdle A bony or cartilaginous arch supporting the lower limbs.

periodization A method of setting up exercise or training programs in periods or blocks of time; for example, if you want to set up a weight-loss exercise program, it might look something like this: (1) weeks 1-3, 30 minutes of cardio three times per week at a low to moderate intensity, (2) weeks 4-8, addition of strength training one time per week and continuation of cardio for 30 minutes three times per week at a moderate intensity, (3) weeks 8-12: strength training two times per week and cardio four times per week, (4) performance of interval training one time per week, a long slow to moderate cardio session two times per week, and 45 minutes of moderate intensity cardio session one time per week. Setting up your exercise program in sets of time with different training tactics during each period of time is called *periodization*.

posture   The carriage of the body as a whole; how one positions the arms and legs. The unconscious and stable structural disposition of the body framework attained over a long period of continuous body movements and patterns.

primary care physician (PCP)   A physician, such as a family practitioner or internist, who is chosen by individuals to provide continuous medical care, trained to treat a wide variety of health-related problems, and responsible for referral of patients to specialists as needed.

pronate   To turn or rotate (the foot) by abduction and eversion so that the inner edge of the sole bears the body's weight.

repetitions   The act of repeating a particular strength exercise a set amount of times. For example, if you perform 10 bicep curls, you've completed 10 repetitions.

resistance bands   Thick bands made of rubber; used for different strength exercises; they are available in several different sizes, colors, and strengths or resistances.

resting metabolic rate   The amount (number) of calories your body needs in a wake and resting state to sustain normal metabolic or physiological functioning; basically the amount (number) of calories your body burns during sedentary activities (e.g., watching TV, reading while sitting down).

retina   The innermost coat of the posterior part of the eyeball that receives the image produced by the lens, is continuous with the optic nerve, and consists of several layers, one of which contains the rods and cones that are sensitive to light.

retinopathy   Any disease or disorder of the retina.

rotator cuff tear   A tear in one of the muscles or tendons of the shoulder. There are four muscles that make up the rotator cuff: supraspinatus, infraspinatus, teres minor, and subscapularis.

scoliosis   A condition of lateral curvature of the spine, which may have just one curve or primary and secondary compensatory curves and may be fixed or mobile.

sets   The number of times a certain number of repetitions are repeated while strength training. For example, if you perform 10 bicep curls three, times, you've completed three sets of 10 repetitions.

Smith machine squat   A form of squat performed on a Smith machine; this machine has a straight bar that is parallel to the floor and connected to two sliding mechanisms that are perpendicular to the horizontal bar.

spondylosis   A medical condition in which there is spinal degeneration and deformity of the joint(s) of two or more vertebrae; commonly occurs with aging. Often, there is herniation of the nucleus pulposus of one or more intervertebral discs and/or formation of osteophytes.

spinal stenosis   A medical condition in which the spinal canal narrows and compresses the spinal cord and nerves; usually due to the natural process of spinal degeneration that occurs with aging. The condition can also sometimes be caused by spinal disc herniation, osteoporosis, or a tumor. Spinal stenosis may affect the cervical spine, the lumbar spine or both.

squat   A strength-training exercise in which a person squats or lowers down, bending at the knees and waist, and then returns to an upright, standing position; squats can be performed with or without weight.

stability ball   A large inflatable ball used primarily to increase core strength.

strength training   Anaerobic exercise intended to increase strength, fitness, and lean muscle mass.

subluxation   Incomplete or partial dislocation.

tendinitis   Inflammation of tendons and of tendon-muscle attachments.

thyroid level   Level of hormones (thyroxine and triiodothyronine) produced by the thyroid gland; has an effect on the regulation of metabolic rate.

tibia   Shin bone; the inner and larger bone of the leg below the knee.

torsion   The act of twisting.

triglycerides   A compound consisting of three molecules of fatty acid converted to glycerol; a neutral fat that is the usual storage form of lipids in the human body.

upper extremity bike (UEB)   A piece of exercise equipment designed to meet the needs of individuals who aren't able to use their lower body for exercise; this equipment offers a cardio workout using the upper body instead of the legs. Essentially designed as a bike using the arms; most UEBs offer wheelchair access.

Valsalva maneuver   Expiratory effort against a closed glottis, which increases pressure within the thoracic cavity and thereby impedes venous return of blood to the heart. The maneuver results in changes in blood pressure and heart rate. Holding your breath and exerting expiratory force should never be done when strength training.

VO2 max testing   See under *fitness assessment*.

waist-to-hip ratio (WHR)   The ratio of the circumference of the waist to that of the hips; a measurement of the proportion by which fat is distributed around the torso. The concept and significance of WHR was first theorized by evolutionary psychologist Dr. Devendra Singh at the University of Texas at Austin in 1993.

weight-bearing activity   An activity that requires weight to be loaded or carried by one or more joints in the body. Walking, running, weight lifting, and squats are all examples of weight-bearing exercises.

GENERAL REFERENCES

American Academy of Orthopedic Surgeons. Available at: http://orthoinfo.aaos.org/topic.cfm?topic=A00032

The American Heritage College Dictionary, 3rd Ed. Boston: Houghton Mifflin, 1993.

Dictionary.com. Available at: http://dictionary.reference.com.

The Free Dictionary. Available at: http://medical-dictionary.thefreedictionary.com

Dorland's Illustrated Medical Dictionary, 28th Ed. Philadelphia: Saunders 1994.

Lab Tests Online. Available at: www.labtestsonline.org/understanding/analytes/a1c/sample.html

Mirriam-Webster Online. Available at: www.merriam-webster.com

Nguyen NT, Silver M, Robinson M, *et al.* Result of a national audit of bariatric surgery performed at academic centers: a 2004 University Health System Consortium Benchmarking Project. *Archives of Surgery* 2006;141:445-449.

WebMD Better Information. Better Health. Available at: ww.webmd.com/cholesterol-management/tc/lipid-panel-topic-overview-management/tc/lipid-panel-topic-overview

Wikipedia. Available at: http://en.wikipedia.org/wiki/Main_Page

Index

A1c 143, 144, 227
Aerobic exercise 48, 51, 62, 71, 78, 85, 94, 95, 106, 158, 227
Acromion 227
Activities of daily living (ADLs) 49, 227
Alcohol 5, 50, 53, 54
Anaerobic exercise 78, 106, 227, 242
Anaerobic threshold 109, 110, 111, 112, 158, 227
Anterior pelvic tilt 125, 227
Arm Ergometer (see also Upper Extremity Bike) 227
Arrhythmias 228
Arthritis 5, 14, 21, 35, 47, 68, 69, 70, 82, 92, 228, 236, 237, 240
Athlete 103, 215, 228,
Back problems 81
    Cervical/upper back 20, 81, 82, 126, 230, 231, 242
    Lumbar/low back 20, 81, 82, 126, 227, 231, 238, 242
Balance 6, 14, 16, 19, 62, 83, 84, 88, 105, 124, 126, 127, 128, 198, 215, 223, 231, 233
Bariatric 26, 35, 56, 92, 93, 94, 95, 177, 184, 219, 228
Bariatric chair 228
Bariatric patient 56
Bariatric surgeon 94, 95, 184
Bariatric surgery 92, 93, 95, 228
    Laparoscopic 94, 219, 238
    Open-cut 94
Benefits of exercise 9, 15
    Health 11, 14, 15, 16, 17, 18, 19, 24, 25, 26, 27, 34, 47, 49, 50, 54, 60, 63, 67, 68, 69, 73, 90, 94, 105, 108, 109, 118, 119, 120, 122, 131, 133, 140, 143, 157, 159, 160, 177, 184, 186, 196, 208, 215, 217, 229, 233, 234, 235
    Weight loss 4, 7, 9, 10, 11, 15, 19, 26, 27, 28, 30, 34, 35, 46, 47, 49, 50, 51, 52, 53, 57, 59, 62, 63, 64, 65, 67, 69, 73, 81, 85, 86, 87, 92, 93, 94, 95, 103, 105, 107, 113, 117, 134, 159, 177, 178, 179, 180, 181, 182, 183, 184, 186, 187, 188, 193, 195, 204, 208, 212, 213, 216, 218, 219, 228, 237
Beta blocker 27, 112, 123, 159, 160, 228,
Blood glucose 50, 51, 66, 72, 73, 74, 75, 76, 141, 143, 144, 212, 229, 232, 234, 235

245

Fasting 143
Blood pressure 11, 15, 27, 54, 79, 80, 87, 112, 118, 119, 120, 129, 159, 199, 208, 209, 212, 229, 236, 243
    Diastolic 79, 80, 119, 120, 229
    Systolic 79, 80, 119, 120, 229
Body bars 229
Body composition 59, 128, 131, 132, 133, 228, 229, 236
Body fat 9, 15, 51, 53, 94, 95, 108, 131, 132, 133, 134, 194, 217, 229, 230, 239
    Body fat testing 132, 230
    Bioelectrical impedance 131, 134, 228
    Hydrostatic weighing 132, 236
    Calipers 131, 230
Body Mass Index (BMI) 11, 84, 128, 129, 130, 209, 212, 217, 229, 237, 239
Body weight 24, 32, 66, 85, 86, 93, 94, 128, 130, 134, 184, 228, 229, 239, 240
Brachial artery 119, 229
Bulging disc 82, 229
Bursitis 92, 229
Callisthenic 75, 230
Cancer 11, 15, 51, 54, 68, 70, 71, 230
    Breast 11, 54, 70, 238
Carotid artery 121, 230
Carbohydrates 39, 48, 50, 51, 52, 53, 58, 94, 103, 104, 105, 106, 109, 158, 182, 234
Cardio 27, 35, 36, 46, 47, 48, 62, 63, 64, 65, 71, 75, 86, 89, 99, 100, 108, 110, 114, 117, 158, 161, 222, 227, 230, 239, 241, 243
Cardiologist 27, 77, 78
Cervical disc disease 82, 230
Children 17, 24, 35, 86, 87, 88, 203, 240
Cholesterol 5, 11, 15, 51, 52, 54, 87, 141, 142, 143, 199, 208, 209, 212, 230, 238
    HDL 11, 15, 54, 142, 208, 230, 231, 238
    LDL 11, 151, 142, 143, 230, 231, 238
    VLDL 142, 143, 230
    Ratios 231
Co-morbidity 231
Comprehensive metabolic panel 142, 231
Compression sleeve 70, 231
Concentric motion 77, 231
Contractures 84
Contraindicated movement 231
Core muscles 81, 126, 231, 238
Degenerative disc disease 82, 231
Diabetes 5, 11, 15, 68, 72, 73, 74, 75, 76, 84, 87, 90, 141, 143, 144, 199, 208, 212, 232
    Gestational 90, 232
    Type I 72-75, 232
    Type II 72, 73, 74, 75, 87, 232
Diet 4, 14, 15, 45, 49-52, 54, 56, 57, 62, 63, 74, 99, 104, 105, 178, 180, 181, 182, 183, 187, 192-194, 200, 209, 212, 215, 218, 219, 228

Recommendations for sample menu 50, 57
Dislocation 79, 92, 232, 242
Dorsiflexion 232
Drop foot 35, 232
Dual adjustable pulley 232
Dumbbells (also see hand weights) 123
Duodenal switch (see also weight loss surgery) 233
Eccentric motion 77, 233
Fat 27, 51, 57, 103, 104, 105, 110, 112, 113, 114, 132, 133
    Burning 9, 10, 15, 27, 48, 63, 64, 95, 103, 105, 106, 107, 110, 112, 113, 114, 120, 237
    The macronutrient 50, 51, 107, 181, 182
Fiber 50, 51, 231
Fitness 26, 27, 29, 33, 45, 117, 133, 159, 161, 162, 163, 223, 224
    Accessories 36, 39, 223
    Clothing 36, 37, 39, 124, 129, 223
    Equipment 17, 24, 30, 31, 32, 34, 35, 36, 41, 99, 100, 110, 131, 144, 148, 152, 155, 161, 163, 223, 224, 227, 229, 243
        Footwear 32, 36, 37
Fitness assessment 60, 61, 161, 163, 233, 243
    1.5-Mile run test 161
    Balance 127, 128, 198, 215, 223, 231, 233
    Flexibility 46, 65, 84, 144, 147, 148, 151, 155
    Muscular strength 47, 48, 59, 69, 126, 127, 128, 164
    Posture 14, 19, 47, 81, 87, 90, 124, 125, 126, 127, 129, 233, 237, 239, 241
    Rockport 1-Mile Walking Test 159, 163
    Strength 16, 26, 27, 48, 49, 52, 64, 70, 77, 80, 86, 87, 100, 164, 168, 171
    VO2 Submax 159
    VO2 Max 109, 110, 112, 158, 159, 160, 163
Fitness Environments 30
    Home 17, 19, 23, 24, 25, 30, 32, 33, 36, 62, 119, 131, 143, 157, 159, 164, 179, 213, 219, 224, 234
    Hotels 31
    Gym/fitness center 27, 30, 33, 34
    Park 23, 30, 32, 33, 37, 62, 66, 85, 159
Fitness professional 19, 20, 23, 24, 25, 26, 27, 28, 45, 63, 64, 77, 89, 92, 99, 100, 109, 158
    Qualifications 21, 30
Flexibility 46, 65, 84, 144, 147, 148, 151, 155
Foot 35, 38, 39, 74, 96, 212, 232, 239, 241
    Care 74, 239
    Type 72, 75
Fracture 88, 234, 240
Frozen shoulder 92, 234
Gastric bypass 56, 92, 212, 214, 215, 217, 219, 234
Gastric sleeve 92, 234

Geriatrics 26, 234
Girth measurements 70, 134, 135, 139, 234
Glucometer 73, 75, 234
Glycemic index 66, 234
Glutes 81, 234
Goals 4, 6, 22, 26, 28, 30, 34, 35, 41, 49, 59, 61, 62, 63, 66, 67, 69, 71, 81, 88, 99, 117, 177, 179, 181, 183, 189, 192, 193, 194, 198, 199, 200, 202, 209, 213, 217, 218
Goniometer 148, 150, 151, 235
Hack squat 89, 164, 165, 166, 167, 168, 242
Hand weights 36
Hamstrings 81, 235
Heart disease 51, 52, 53, 54, 77, 142, 199, 208, 234
Heart rate 27, 36, 39, 40, 63, 64, 75, 107, 109, 110, 111, 112, 113, 114, 118, 120, 121, 122, 123, 124, 159, 160, 161, 224, 228, 230, 234, 235, 236, 240, 243
    Ambient 120, 122, 235
    Maximal 60, 123, 158, 225, 233, 235
    Recovery 90, 120, 123, 124, 222, 235
    Resting 10, 48, 49, 80, 104, 105, 112, 113, 114, 120, 121, 122, 158, 209, 213, 219, 222, 235, 237, 240, 241
Heart rate monitor 39, 40, 107, 120, 121, 159, 160, 161, 224, 230
Hernia 171, 230
Herniated disc 230

Hip 19, 78, 79, 81, 125, 128, 139, 140, 151, 236, 243
Hip flexors 81, 236
Hip replacement 79, 230
Hiss/Compress exercise 91
Hypertension 79, 80, 84, 119, 120, 228, 230
Hypertrophic cardiomyopathy 78, 230
Hypoglycemia 72, 75, 76, 234, 236
Hypothyroidism 141, 144, 237
Impingement 92, 237
Indirect calorimetry 49, 60, 109, 158, 209, 237
Insulin 72, 73, 74, 75, 199, 232, 236
Interval training 64, 108, 236, 241
Karvonen method 112, 113, 114, 230, 237
Kegal exercises 91, 237
Knee replacement x, 78, 79, 237
Kyphosis 120, 237
Lab work 118, 208, 142
Lap band 92, 237
Lat pulldown 238
Lifestyle change 3, 5, 31, 59
Lipid panel 142, 238
Lordosis 126, 238
Low-impact activity 79, 238
Lumpectomy 70, 238
Lymphedema 70, 231, 238
Magic pill 14, 15
Mastectomy 70, 238
Metabolism 10, 25, 27, 49, 52, 57, 72, 73, 74, 95, 101, 104, 134, 144, 179, 181, 185, 219, 222, 227, 232, 237, 238

Index

Metabolize 48, 95, 104, 105, 109, 134, 158, 238
Minerals 52, 53
    Essential 50, 51, 54, 73, 101, 133
    Non-essential 54
Mitochondria 10, 238
Multiple sclerosis 68, 82, 238
Muscular dystrophy 68, 83, 84, 239
Myocardial infarction 78, 239
Neuropathy 73, 74, 75, 239
Neutral alignment 124, 125, 165, 239
Obesity IX, XIII, 11, 14, 15, 18, 28, 51, 54, 84, 85, 86, 87, 92, 94, 95, 101, 130, 131, 140, 173, 177, 180, 182, 184, 187, 212, 219, 228, 234, 238, 239, 240
    Class I 85, 131, 239
    Class II 85, 131, 239
    Morbid 85, 92, 101, 187, 212, 217, 234, 240
One-rep maximum 87, 240
Osteopenia 88, 89, 240
Osteophytes 240, 242
Osteoporosis 14, 16, 49, 68, 88, 89, 240, 242
Obstacles 4, 8, 16, 17, 61, 183, 194
    Overcoming 4, 17
Over training 63, 122, 213, 215, 240
Pacemaker 39
Pediatrics 26, 240
Pelvic girdle 125, 240
Periodization 28, 240, 241
Posture 14, 19, 47, 81, 89, 90, 124, 125, 126, 127, 129, 233, 237, 239, 241

Primary care physician (PCP) 27, 241
Pronate 241
Protein 48, 50, 52, 53, 56, 57, 66, 74, 100, 104, 105, 107, 108, 181, 215
Repetitions 25, 49, 64, 65, 70, 77, 80, 84, 86, 89, 90, 91, 165, 168, 171, 241, 242
Resistance bands 24, 36, 100, 241
Resting metabolic rate (RMR) 10, 49
Retinopathy 73, 76, 242
Rotator cuff tear 242
Scoliosis 84, 126, 242
Sets 49, 64, 65, 70, 77, 80, 86, 89, 90, 241, 242
Shoulder injury 92
Sick 19, 20, 22, 33, 59, 117, 217
Smith machine 89, 242
Spondylosis 82, 242
Spinal stenosis 82, 231, 242
Squat 89, 164, 165, 166, 167, 168, 242
    Chair 31, 63, 83, 84, 96, 99, 100, 128, 164, 165, 166, 167, 168, 200, 228
    Smith machine 89, 242
Stability ball 31, 242
Subluxation 92, 242
Sunglasses 36, 39, 224
Tendonitis 92
Thyroid level 243
Torsion 82, 243
Triglycerides 11, 15, 142, 143, 173, 212, 230, 238, 243
Upper Extremity Bike (UEB) 243
Valsalva maneuver 243

Vitamins 51, 54, 131
VO2 max 109, 110, 112, 158, 159, 160, 163, 173
    VO2 max testing (see also indirect calorimetry) 109, 158
Waist-to-hip ratio 243
Water 33, 36, 38, 39, 40, 50, 52, 53, 54, 58, 66, 69, 70, 76, 105, 121, 132, 134, 190, 201, 203, 229, 230
Weight bearing 70, 101

Weight-loss surgery IX, X, 50, 56, 92, 94, 95, 134, 178, 181, 182, 184, 185, 187, 215, 216, 217, 219, 228, 233, 237
    Duodenal switch 92, 233
    Gastric bypass (RNY) 56, 92, 212, 214, 215, 217, 219, 234
    Gastric sleeve 92, 234
    Lap band 92, 237

Made in the USA